Healing
FOODS

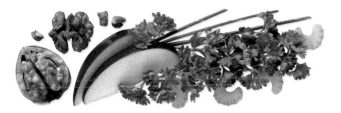

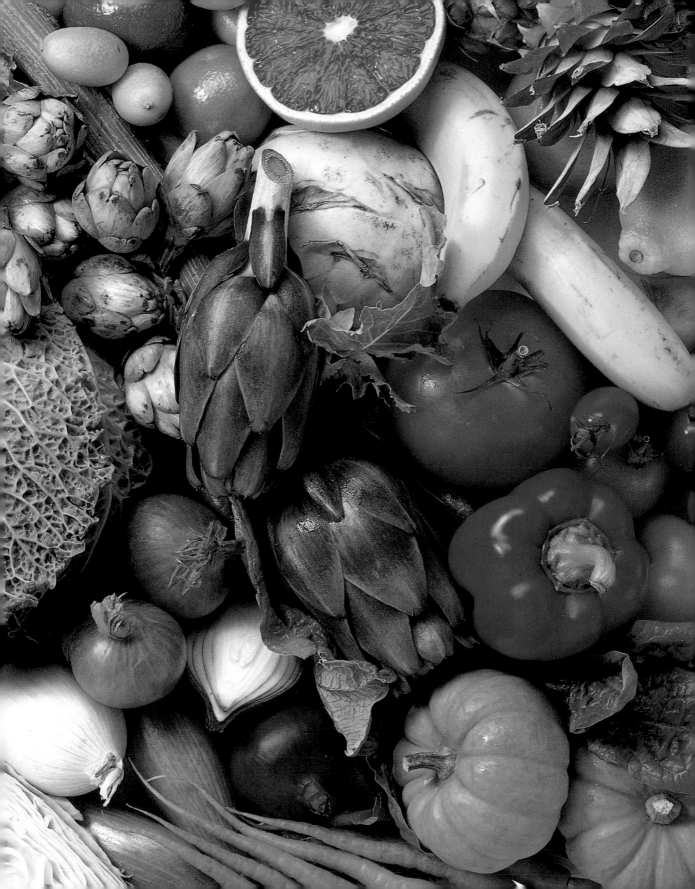

Healing FOODS

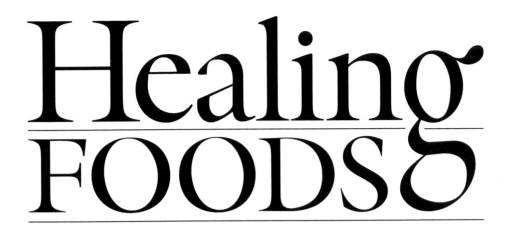

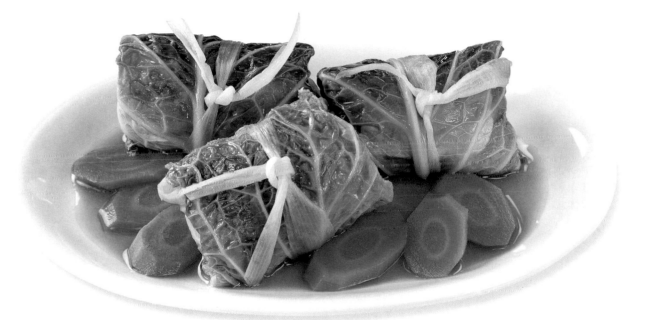

MIRIAM POLUNIN

DK
DK PUBLISHING, INC.

A DK PUBLISHING BOOK

Project Editor Blanche Sibbald

Editor Annabel Martin

Art Editor John Dinsdale

Designer Laura Jackson

Senior Editors Rosie Pearson, Penny Warren

US Editors Laaren Brown, Constance Novis

Managing Editors Fay Franklin, Mary Ling

Managing Art Editor Virginia Walter

Photography
Andy Crawford, Steve Gorton

Food Photography Andrew Whittuck

DTP Designers
Suzy Dittmar, Paul Wood

Production Manager Maryann Rogers

•

Dedicated to my son Joe Vester

First American Edition, 1997
2 4 6 8 10 9 7 5 3 1

Published in the United States by DK Publishing Inc.,
95 Madison Avenue, New York, New York 10016
Visit us on the World Wide Web at http://www.dk.com

Library of Congress Cataloging-in-Publication Data

Polunin, Miriam.
    Healing Foods / by Miriam Polunin. -- 1st American ed.
    p.   cm.
    Includes index.
    ISBN 0-7894-1456-2
    1. Nutrition--Popular works.   2. Diet therapy--Popular works.
I. Title.
RA784.P645   1996
613.2--dc20
                                                96-30980
                                                CIP

Reproduced in Singapore by Colourscan
Printed and bound in Singapore by Star Standard Industries

CONTENTS

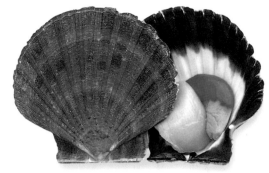

INTRODUCTION 6

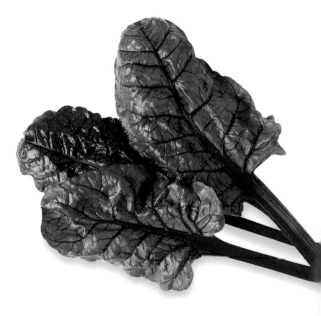

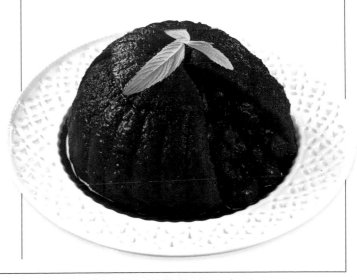

INTRODUCTION

MORE THAN 2,000 YEARS AGO, Hippocrates wrote: *"Each one of the substances of a man's diet acts upon his body and changes it in some way, and upon these changes his whole life depends, whether he be in health, in sickness, or convalescent."*

Over the past decade, research into the effects of food on health has given a welcome new look to healthy eating. The message is that eating more of many foods we find attractive is just as important to our well-being as avoiding too much fat or sugar.

Of the thousands of plants and animals around us, humans only eat a few hundred species. These are foods that over the centuries have proved themselves as foods that work for man, and that's probably why we like their taste. Current research is confirming that many of the colors, smells, textures, and flavors we find attractive in traditional foods are not just nature's garnishes. Features such as the brilliant colors of carrots or tomatoes, or the savory smell of onions, come from substances in food that can strongly benefit our health – both known vitamins and minerals, and more recently explored substances with special properties.

Since the 1950s, large-scale diet surveys, hospital trials, and laboratory tests have contributed evidence that, even in affluent communities, variations in eating habits are a main factor in disease. Food research is never simple, because there are so many elements in health. But gradually, international agreement has emerged among nutrition experts on the kind of eating habits that give us the best chance of good health. Their advice is not just to eat less fat or more fiber, but to eat more of certain foods that, for reasons not yet understood, are turning out to be positively protective. The evidence that we benefit by eating more of many foods dispels the negativity that often surrounds healthy eating. Constant self-denial saps many people's pleasure in food, and may lead to a sense of rebellion in which they give up their efforts to eat for health. However, a healthy diet based on eating *more* of many foods can restore *joie de vivre*. It's also an essential part of countering the eating pattern that has made people in developed countries so vulnerable to illnesses such as coronary heart disease, stroke, diabetes, and some cancers.

If we value our health, we must adjust to a less-active lifestyle. Daily activity is crucial to good health, but most people do not burn the number of calories that was almost universal before cars and other energy-saving devices. We must also adapt to being surrounded by easily available high-fat food that appeals to tastes inherited from our forebears. Eating more of the protective foods enables us to match modern needs by taking in less fat and fewer calories, while still enjoying food and obtaining enough nutrients.

This book presents the positive side of healthy eating. In addition to information about choosing the balance of foods now recommended by nutrition experts worldwide, there are profiles of 50 bonus foods with outstanding nutritional value and special health-helping properties. The profiles combine information from scientific studies, including nutritional research and probing into less-known properties, with traditional healing uses and information on how to enjoy the foods in a Western-style diet.

In this book, scientific information has had to be condensed and simplified, which can give the misleading impression that it is both more straightforward and certain than it is. Scientific knowledge of what food can do for us is far from complete. In particular, we don't know how much reducing a risk factor, such as raised blood cholesterol, will lower the risk of the related illness for a particular individual. The view I take is that current research offers many useful pointers for practical action against common diseases. Even the best-tested uses of food for prevention and healing will not work for everyone, but, at worst, you will widen your eating habits and improve your nutritional status. After all, one of the strongest messages to come from research is that eating a wide variety of food is valuable for health.

"Optimum nutrition" is now a possibility. Those of us who are lucky enough to have ample food available can enjoy eating and choose foods that help prevent and treat illness and enhance well-being. You don't have to be a fanatic: every move in the right direction counts. The quest is not so much for extra years in our life, but for extra life in our years.

Miriam Polunin

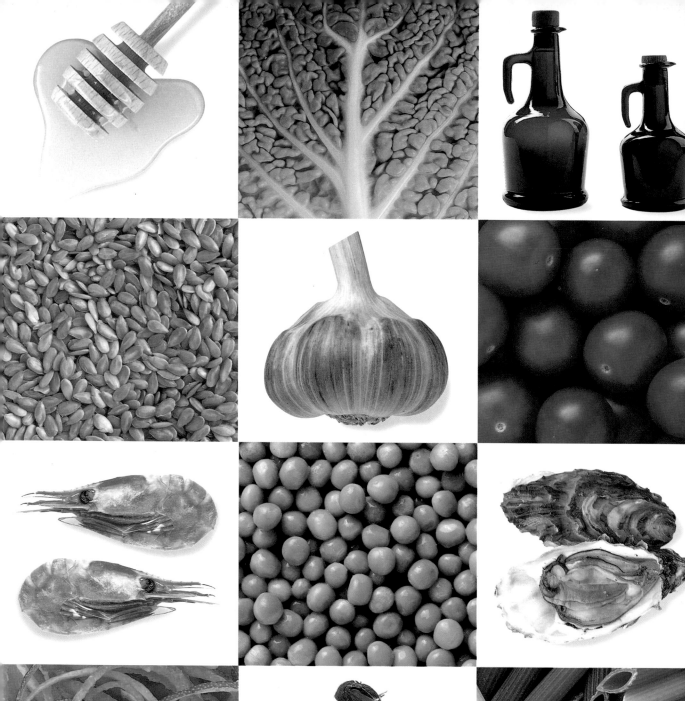

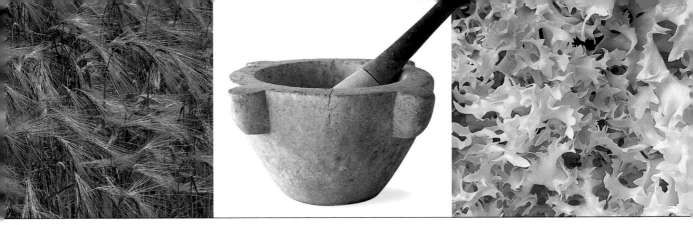

THE BALANCE OF HEALTH

An introduction to food as a positive force for health and well-being.
Advice on the balance of foods we need and guidance
on the special substances that make certain foods particularly
valuable, to help you choose and enjoy food with confidence.

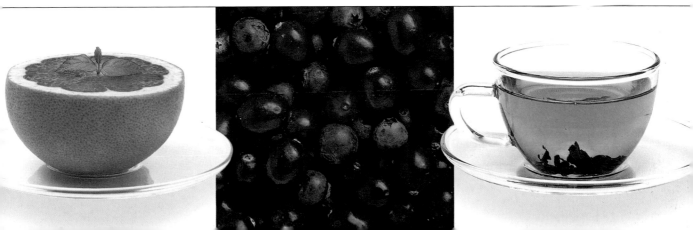

FOOD AS MEDICINE

EVERY CULTURE THROUGHOUT history has used food both to prevent and to treat illness: Chinese emperors employed Imperial dietitians as far back as the 4th century BCE, and ancient Egyptian physicians correctly recommended eating liver as a way of treating night blindness. Industrialized countries have passed through a period when healing through diet has been labeled ineffective or worse. Now, there is a renewed acceptance of the vital role food plays in maintaining health. A major factor in changing attitudes has been the ability, thanks to computers, to compare the eating habits of large numbers of people with their risk of disease. These surveys have proved how much food matters in disease prevention and have led to research into the effects of many individual foods and diet patterns on health.

❖ TRADITIONAL CURES ❖

THE TRADITION OF FOOD MEDICINES

The traditional uses of food as medicine are based on observation and continual assessment over a long period of time. The effects of eating certain foods were noted and remembered, and gradually a community would acquire knowledge that could be used to enhance its health and survival.

The distinction between "food" and "medicine" might have seemed strange to our early ancestors: the plants and animals around them were their only resources, and had to serve all purposes. With times of hunger and illness spurring on experimentation, our early ancestors would have tried almost everything around them for its food and medicinal value. While in recent times we have laughed at the superstitions and rites that often went with this traditional knowledge, it is unreasonable to dismiss the whole tradition of food medicines.

The scientific examination of several traditional food medicines has been reassuring: cabbage does indeed have the protective properties that the Romans wrote about, and pumpkin seeds can help prostate health, as European herbal tradition holds. But how do we assess traditional food uses that have little or no scientific backing? Key questions are how long and how widely has the food been used medicinally. Fennel, for instance, has been employed as a food medicine from ancient Greece and Rome to medieval Britain and modern China. Drawn by these wide-ranging uses, modern researchers are becoming increasingly interested in looking more closely at the effects of a particular food. Food medicines have another advantage over synthesized drugs because although "natural" does not always mean safe, our traditional foods have been tested for longer and by far more people.

Native Americans
The first European settlers arriving in North America were introduced to many new foods by the Native Americans. Early sailors quickly learned that cranberries were helpful for scurvy.

❖ SCIENTIFIC RESEARCH ❖

RESEARCH INTO THE HEALTH BENEFITS OF FOOD

Understanding the effects of eating a particular food is an exciting area of research, with many unanswered questions. We do not know if the health benefits of many foods are nutritional, preventing or relieving a disease by giving the body the nutrients it needs to thrive and fight off illness; physical, due to elements in food such as fiber; or pharmacological, due to active substances that may be potentially therapeutic or protective, see p. 21. In many cases, results will be the result of the combined effects of several constituents. Testing single substances from food – for example, beta-carotene from vegetables – has often shown different effects from tests of the whole food.

Scientific interest into how particular foods or eating habits can prevent, cause, or treat many illnesses is now intense. Some foods and nutrients have been investigated far more than others. For example, there have been about a thousand scientific papers published on oily fish, but a mere handful on honey. Hundreds of studies have examined the effects of different levels of iron in the body, but so far, very few have looked at zinc in this manner because no reliable way has been found yet of judging what body level of zinc is desirable.

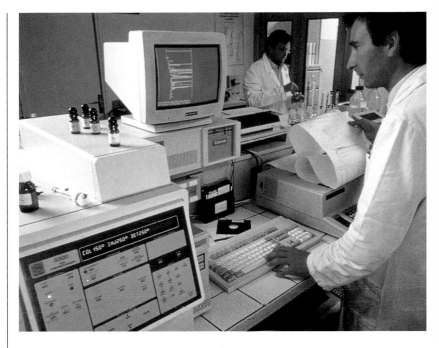

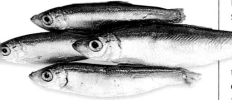

Whitebait
The benefits of oily fish have been widely studied. In general, money for research into food is scarce because it will not lead to a patented product.

TYPES OF SCIENTIFIC RESEARCH

Lack of scientific evidence for a food or nutrient does not necessarily prove that it has less benefit. Some foods are less closely examined for reasons of cost, commercial possibilities, ethical problems, practical difficulties of analysis or resources if a very long trial is required, or simply because the subject has not attracted the interest of researchers – yet.

Scientific evidence varies greatly in its strength, depending on the kind of research that has been done. For example, a link between food and illness is strongest if it is based on several studies, including highly controlled experiments in which two groups of similar people are compared. One group will eat a measured amount of the food being tested, and the other group will be given a placebo. The most convincing "double blind" trials

High-tech research *Large-scale diet surveys rely on computers to compare dietary records with health results, sometimes following a group of volunteers over many years.*

then repeat the test, swapping the groups.

Studies based on comparisons using large groups of people are more convincing than ones using small numbers. Studying what ill people recall eating in the time before they were diagnosed with an illness (when their eating habits may already have been affected by the disease) has less impact than recording everything a large number of people eat for a week, and then waiting some years to compare that with their later health.

Research on groups of people can never prove that changing the diet will protect or heal a particular individual because there are so many factors in illness. Yet science increasingly confirms the power of foods to improve our chances of attaining good health.

THE BASIC HEALTHY DIET

EVERY TIME YOU TAKE a mouthful of food, you are refueling the most clever chemical mechanism known: the human body. Food and water provide the fuel of vital nutrients that enable the body to function. Fighting off invading harmful bacteria, balancing the fluid level so that it stays stable even on a very hot day, and millions of other processes all need the chemicals from food in order to work efficiently. Some foods have more to offer than others, but you do not have to give up the foods you most enjoy for the sake of your health: any food can fit into a healthy style of eating at least occasionally. It is the combinations and quantities you choose that are important to help protect your well-being.

FRUITS AND VEGETABLES
Eat a wide variety of fruits and vegetables in generous amounts. Green leafy vegetables and yellow, orange, and red fruits and vegetables are especially beneficial.

THE MAIN FOOD GROUPS
The circle of food, *right*, is divided into segments showing the proportions of the main food groups that make up a basic healthy diet. Several governments have produced pictorial food guides like this, to make it easier to choose a healthy balance of food. It is not necessary to follow a strict regimen or to work out exact percentages of different foods to eat: the human body is amazingly efficient at adapting to slightly higher or lower intakes. Although the total amount eaten will vary according to energy needs, this balance of foods from the different groups is desirable for almost everyone from the age of five.

MEAT, FISH, AND PROTEIN ALTERNATIVES
Consume moderate amounts from this group, which includes meat, fish, poultry, eggs, legumes, shellfish, nuts, and seeds.

SUGARY AND HIGH-FAT FOODS
Foods high in sugar or fat are best eaten sparingly. These include foods such as medium and high-fat cheeses, butter, margarine, and cooking oils, as well as cookies and other sweetened foods.

STARCHY FOODS

Eat starchy foods in generous amounts. These include bread, pasta, potatoes, yams, sweet potatoes, and cereal grains such as oats, barley, rice, millet, corn, and kasha. Choose versions with little added fat or sugar whenever possible.

DAIRY FOODS

Enjoy dairy foods in moderate amounts. Best choices include skim milk and nonfat milk, low-fat varieties of yogurt, fromage frais, pot cheese, cottage cheese, cream cheese, and farmer cheese.

HOW MUCH TO EAT

International consensus about what proportion each of the main food groups should take up in the diet is as follows:

STARCHY FOODS

Starchy foods like bread, cereal grains, and potatoes are the foundation of a balanced diet. Most people in developed countries would benefit from eating about 50% more of these foods, especially unrefined versions, which provide more fiber, vitamins, and minerals.

FRUITS AND VEGETABLES

Try to eat at least 5 servings of fruits and vegetables a day, which amounts to at least 14oz (400g), not including potatoes, sweet potatoes, or yams, eaten as part of the starchy foods intake. Fresh or frozen produce is best. Small amounts of fruit juice, canned fruits (preferably in unsweetened juice), and dried fruits can contribute to the 5-a-day servings.

MEAT, FISH, AND PROTEIN ALTERNATIVES

It is advisable to eat fish at least twice a week, including at least 1 serving of oily fish. Eating 1oz (30g) of legumes (dry weight), nuts, or seeds a day is desirable. Except for these, it is best to choose lower-fat versions as often as possible. For most people eating a Western-style diet, it is a good idea to eat a little less from this group and more starchy foods, fruits, and vegetables.

DAIRY FOODS

Eat in moderation and choose low-fat versions as often as possible. Fat levels in "low-fat" dairy foods vary considerably: look for soft cheese with a 7–8% fat level and yogurt with a 1–2% fat level. Low-fat yogurt or low-fat sour cream are good replacements for higher-fat cream, such as sour cream and heavy cream.

SUGARY AND HIGH-FAT FOODS

Although this group includes some foods such as cheese and sunflower oil that are valuable in small amounts, most foods high in sugar or fat are low in food value for their calorie level and are best eaten sparingly. These include butter and margarine, cream, fried food, potato chips, candies, chocolate, and most cakes, pastries, and cookies. Eating less from this food group allows you to eat more starchy foods and fruits and vegetables without gaining weight.

WHAT'S IN FOOD

THE ELEMENTS FOUND IN food fall into four main groups: macronutrients, which are needed in substantial amounts for energy and include carbohydrates, fats, and protein; micronutrients, which are vital but needed in only tiny amounts and include two essential fatty acids, vitamins, and minerals; fibrous carbohydrates, which cannot be used for energy; and, finally, water. Food also contains many other substances that can affect our health, for better or worse. Some of these have special properties that may be valuable in protecting health, even if they are not essential, as some may yet turn out to be. There is a great deal about our sophisticated nutrition system that we do not yet understand. Luckily, we can obtain the food elements we need without that knowledge by following the Basic Healthy Diet, pp. 12–13.

❖ CARBOHYDRATES ❖

TYPES OF CARBOHYDRATES

Carbohydrates are our main source of energy. The simplest forms are sugars – for example, glucose and fructose – which combined make sucrose, the common crystal sugar. You are unlikely to eat large amounts of sugar from natural sources, such as fruits and vegetables, because it is diluted with water and fiber.

Compounds of several sugars are called complex carbohydrates. The most common of these is starch, found mainly in starchy foods such as bread, pasta, and potatoes, as well as in other foods like legumes and less-ripe bananas. During digestion, the body splits most carbohydrates back into simple sugars and needs to produce insulin to absorb them to use as energy.

Fiber and resistant starch are the names of some carbohydrates that the body cannot fully digest.

VITAL FOR GOOD HEALTH

Starchy foods, such as bread, pasta, rice and other grains, potatoes, and yams, are our main source of complex carbohydrates. These foods also supply a substantial amount of protein, vitamins, minerals, and fiber, with little fat. Starchy foods are the staple diet worldwide, yet many people wrongly believe that they are less valuable to the body than protein-rich foods.

For good health, most nutrition experts recommend that starchy foods should supply about half the daily calorie intake. Most of us enjoy these foods but, in the last 50 years, the amount of starchy foods eaten by people in Western countries has plunged, so that they now supply only about 30% of the daily calorie intake.

Communities that eat little starchy food generally have higher rates of heart disease, stroke, obesity, many forms of cancer, diabetes, gallstones, and bowel disorders than communities that eat more of these foods. This link may be because people who eat more starchy foods generally eat less fat. But starchy foods also supply fiber, and starch itself may have protective properties, which are now being researched.

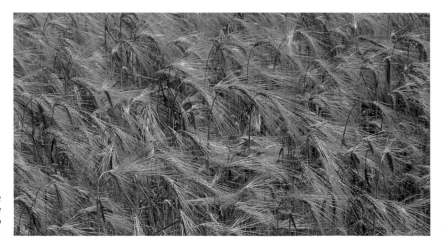

Field of barley *Cereal grains are cheaper than animal foods, not because they are of less value for our health, but because they require much less energy to produce.*

AN IMPORTANT PART OF LOW-FAT EATING

Eating more starchy foods is almost essential if you want to eat less fat and sugar. Every time you avoid eating some fat or sugar you eat fewer calories. For example, if you avoid eating 1 tablespoon of fat you skip or miss 135 calories. Eating 4 teaspoons less sugar saves about 80 calories. Unless you wish to lose weight, you need to recover that energy in another form. Eating extra fruits and vegetables will help, but most contain so few calories for their bulk that you are liable to feel over-full if they are your only way of replacing calories. You could eat more low-fat dairy foods, meat, or fish, but eating more protein than you need has drawbacks, see p. 20, and is expensive. Starchy foods are the enjoyable and affordable answer.

Calories in food *Just a few slices of a high-fat food, such as salami, provide the same number of calories as a much larger and more filling portion of a starchy food, such as rice. Calories eaten as starch rather than as fat are less likely to be stored as body fat.*

STARCHY FOODS CAN HELP WEIGHT CONTROL

A major advantage of eating more starchy foods is that they are much lower in fat than many other foods. Starchy foods are also more filling than the same number of calories eaten in a fatty form. For example, a substantial 2oz (55g) serving of rice (dry weight, white or brown) provides 200 calories, while the same number of calories is provided by a mere 1½ oz (40g) of high-fat salami. This is because 1g of fat has 9 calories, compared with 3.75 calories in 1g of carbohydrate.

Starchy foods make it easier to satisfy your appetite without eating too many calories. Eating more starchy foods and a little less fat and sugar each day aids weight control. Furthermore, if not used up in activity, calories eaten in the form of starch are less readily stored as body fat than calories eaten as fat. This is because it is harder work for the body (using up more calories) to convert surplus carbohydrate into body fat than it is to turn excess fat we consume into body fat.

CHOOSING STARCHY FOODS

Starchy foods lose their advantages if they have a high level of added sugar or fat. For example, a breakfast cereal with a little bit of added sugar is still helpful, but the high sugar and fat content of most cakes and cookies outweighs their starchy or fibrous value.

Most bread gets 7–10% of its calories from fat, but short dough pastry gets 56% of its calories from fat. Pastry, most sweet and savory biscuits, sugary breakfast cereals, potato chips, french fries, cookies, and cakes are foods to eat sparingly. But there are still many popular starchy foods to enjoy, including some unexpected items such as currant buns, pancakes, scones, and rice pudding. When eating starchy foods like bread or pasta, use lower-fat spreads or pasta sauces. The more starchy food you eat, the more you rely on it for nutrients, so it becomes important to choose mainly unrefined versions of starchy foods such as whole grains, which are much higher in vitamins and minerals than the refined versions.

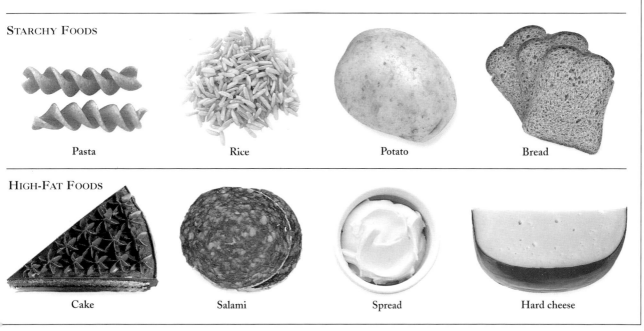

STARCHY FOODS

Pasta   Rice   Potato   Bread

HIGH-FAT FOODS

Cake   Salami   Spread   Hard cheese

❖ TYPES OF FIBER ❖

There are two main groups of fiber, insoluble and soluble, and both kinds are needed for good health. Soluble fiber is found primarily in oats, legumes, nuts, seeds, fruits, and vegetables. Cereal grains, especially unrefined whole grains, are the main source of insoluble fiber.

SOLUBLE FIBER LEADS TO STEADIER ENERGY

Rather than speeding up the transit time of food waste, soluble fiber slows down the rate of digestion in the stomach, providing a steadier flow of energy. Eating plenty of foods rich in soluble fiber has also been shown to encourage healthier blood fat levels and to help reduce blood cholesterol.

Oatmeal

Sugar and low-fiber starchy foods are digested more rapidly than foods high in soluble fiber. When you eat them, the level of sugar in your blood rises rapidly and is quickly available as energy to be used or stored. But the higher the rise in blood sugar, the faster the fall. Carbohydrate foods rich in soluble fiber or resistant starch give a gentler rise, which lasts longer. People vary in how easily they cope with ups and downs in blood sugar. But for many, especially diabetics or those who are overweight, steadier blood sugar levels have major advantages: they help steady energy levels and can also help stabilize mood.

Stable blood sugar levels make less demand on the insulin mechanism, which is needed to convert sugar from the blood into usable energy. This in turn may help weight control by delaying the return of hunger, either real or in reaction to a drop in mood as blood sugar falls.

Recent research suggests a link between high body levels of insulin and several disorders, notably abdominal obesity, higher levels of blood fats, and higher levels of estrogen, a sign of increased risk of breast cancer.

Foods rich in soluble fiber *such as dried apricots, oatmeal, and lentils tend to raise blood sugar more gently than foods high in sugar, giving steadier energy.*

Dried apricots

Split red lentils

Even among high-fiber foods, some raise blood sugar much more sharply than others. Not all reasons for this are known, although foods with less sugar or more soluble fiber, or foods composed of larger particles, tend to raise blood sugar less. So, a less ripe banana raises blood sugar more gently than a ripe banana, and apples more mildly than apple juice. Researchers have produced "blood sugar ratings" for foods, see p. 91. These compare the average blood sugar surge after eating each food with the level after eating the same amount of carbohydrate from glucose.

INSOLUBLE FIBER SPEEDS THE PASSAGE OF WASTE

By increasing the bulk of the feces, insoluble fiber helps food waste pass through the digestive tract quickly and easily. Eating plenty of cereal grains not only prevents constipation, which is associated with hemorrhoids and an increased risk of bowel diseases, but also helps the body remove harmful substances faster. Research is in progress to establish if eating more insoluble fiber and resistant starch (a carbohydrate that resists digestion) reduces the high risk of serious bowel disorders, including colon and bowel cancer, in Western countries.

Unrefined whole grains are important for insoluble fiber. The outer layers, which contain almost all the fiber, also contain most of the vitamins and minerals. Try to eat unrefined whole grains and unpeeled fruits and vegetables as often as possible.

There is no advantage in eating very large amounts of insoluble fiber, especially in the form of wheat bran. The fiber in wheat bran, along with a substance called phytic acid (which is reduced in breadmaking), make it harder for the body to absorb zinc, iron, and calcium from food. Too much fiber can make you feel bloated.

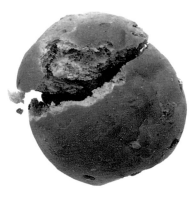

Whole-grain bread *It is better to eat insoluble fiber in whole-wheat and whole-grain breads than in bran cereals, which reduce mineral absorption.*

IMPROVING YOUR DAILY INTAKE OF FIBER

Most people living in industrialized countries would benefit from eating more insoluble and soluble fiber. A typical Western intake is about ¹/₂ oz (12–18g) a day, compared with expert advice to eat ¹/₂–1oz (16–28g) a day, according to our calorie intake. You do not have to eat bran or unrefined cereal grains exclusively in order to obtain a good daily intake of fiber.

A High-Fiber Menu

		Approximate fiber g
BREAKFAST	2 x 1oz (25g) slices of whole-wheat toast	3.0
or	1oz (30g) whole-grain breakfast cereal with any kind of milk	
	5¼ oz (150g) apple, unpeeled weight	2.7
MIDMORNING	6oz (175g) banana, unpeeled weight	1.2
LUNCH	1 sandwich made with 2½ oz (75g) whole-wheat bread, excluding filling	4.5
	3½ oz (100g) coleslaw	1.6
SNACK	1 oat bran muffin	2.0
EVENING MEAL	10fl oz (300ml) cream of tomato soup	1.5
	1 serving of roast chicken	0.0
	1¾ oz (50g) brown rice, dry weight	1.0
	3½ oz (100g) peas, fresh or frozen	5.0
	1 slice of apple pie, with whole-wheat crust	4.4
TOTAL		26.9

A Low-Fiber Menu

		Approximate fiber g
BREAKFAST	2 x 1oz (25g) slices of white toast	1.0
	1oz (30g) cornflakes with any kind of milk	0.3
MIDMORNING	1oz (30g) sweet, whole-wheat cookie	0.7
LUNCH	1 sandwich made with 2½ oz (75g) white bread, excluding filling	1.4
	5¼ oz (150g) apple, unpeeled weight	2.7
SNACK	1 x 1oz (30g) bag of potato chips	1.6
	1 x 1¾ oz (50g) chocolate bar	0.4
EVENING MEAL	10fl oz (300ml) chicken soup	trace
	1 serving of grilled fish	0.0
	1¾ oz (50g) white pasta, dry weight	1.5
	7oz (200g) green salad	1.8
	1 slice of cheesecake	0.6
TOTAL		12.0

THE POOR NUTRITIONAL VALUE OF SUGAR

Although sugar contains the same 3.75 calories per gram as other carbohydrates, it is the only food that provides no fiber, vitamins, minerals, or other useful nutrients. International nutritional advice is to eat as little added sugar as possible, on average under 2oz (60g) a day for an adult. The body does not need sugar, and it is not superior to other foods for energy, except after prolonged heavy exercise.

Sugar is not particularly fattening, and a little does no harm. Sugar that is naturally present in foods such as fruits and milk does not need to be limited. But most Westerners "waste" about 9–14% of their calories eating around 1¾–2½ oz (50–75g) a day of added sugars, for instance in ready-made foods, sweetened drinks, or homemade cakes. For example, a large soda pop contains over 1½ oz (40g) of sugar and a 2oz (60g) chocolate bar supplies 1oz (30g).

Surveys show that children are especially likely to eat more than average amounts of sugar, and are also more susceptible to tooth decay. In industrialized societies, most people's calorie needs have fallen significantly, but our needs for nutrients have not. If we are to maintain our nutrient intake while eating less food, it is less and less practical to use up calories on sugar, which provides no nutrients.

Sugary drinks and foods *such as cola drinks and chocolate are best consumed seldom, or not at all.*

❖ FATS ❖

TYPES OF FAT

Almost all of the fat in food consists of fatty acids, which are saturated, monounsaturated, or polyunsaturated, terms derived from their chemical composition (see below). Although fatty foods contain fatty acids from all 3 groups, saturated fats predominate in farmed meat and dairy foods, while plants contain mainly unsaturated fats, and fish and shellfish contain almost only poly-unsaturated fats. Another kind of fatty acid, known as trans fatty acid, occurs naturally in small amounts, but is mainly a result of hydrogenation, the deliberate saturating of unsaturated fats to harden them for use in processed foods, such as cookies or spreads.

Cholesterol is a waxy substance found in animal foods and is related to fat. It is just as high in some lean foods as it is in fatty foods.

CHEMICAL COMPOSITION

There are 26 common fatty acids, with short or long chains of carbon atoms, each with a space for a hydrogen atom. If every space is occupied, the fatty acid is saturated; if 2 hydrogen positions are unfilled, a double bond will occur between 2 carbon atoms and the fatty acid is monounsaturated; if 4 or more hydrogen spaces are unfilled, more double bonds will occur and the fatty acid is polyunsaturated. In food, fats are grouped into triglycerides, combinations of 3 fatty acids with a unit of glycerol.

WHY WE NEED SOME FAT

To enjoy a wide choice of food, eating some fat is necessary. Most foods contain some fat. Fat is the only source of essential and other important fatty acids. Most vitamin E is in fatty foods, and fat is needed to absorb vitamins A, D, E, and K. People who lack vitamin D,

obtained by the exposure of skin to sunlight, need to eat certain fats containing this vitamin. Animal fat also supplies vitamin A, although the body can produce all it needs from carotenes in vegetables and fruits. Although the Western-style diet contains a high level of fat, it can still fail to supply enough of these vitamins. For example, many fatty foods contain no vitamin D.

DANGERS OF TOO MUCH FAT

Eating too much fat has many adverse effects, depending on our constitution, lifestyle, and the type of fat we choose. Eating fat of any kind beyond our needs unbalances our diet, using up the calories we need to "spend" on eating more starchy foods, fruits, and vegetables.

Too much fat easily leads to excess weight, increasing the risk of illnesses. Too much saturated fat is a strong risk factor for heart disease and stroke. Fat supplies 9 calories per gram, compared with about 4 calories per gram of protein or carbohydrate, and excess calories are more readily stored as body fat when eaten as fat. For those who need to lose weight, eating less fat is the best way to reduce calorie intake without losing necessary nutrients.

Fats vary in their effects. We are strongly advised to eat less saturated fat. Generally, the more solid a fat is at room temperature, the higher the level of saturated and trans fatty acids. Nutritional experts believe that reducing fat intake, from the typical present level of 40% of total calories to 30–35%, by eating less saturated and trans fatty acids, makes a substantial difference in the risk of disease. For most people, this is a moderate change. For a woman eating about 1,800 calories a day, it means reducing fat from about 80g a day to 60–70g: a drop of less than ⅔ oz. For a man

eating about 2,400 calories, it means reducing fat from 106g to 80–93g: a drop of about ½–1oz. Most of this drop can be made by eating less saturated and trans fats. The aim is to reduce these to 10–11% of calories, about ¾ oz (22g) a day for a typical woman and 1oz (28g) for a typical man.

CHOLESTEROL

Cholesterol is a form of fat that the body needs for several functions: for example, it is needed in enzyme systems and the manufacture of hormones. The body can produce all the cholesterol it needs and does not require the cholesterol we eat in animal foods.

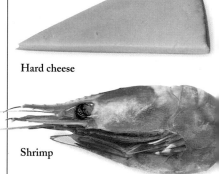

Hard cheese

Shrimp

Cholesterol facts
For most people, foods that are high in total fat and saturated fat, such as hard cheese, stimulate a rise in blood cholesterol level more than foods that contain high amounts of cholesterol but are low in fat, such as shrimp and other shellfish.

A high level of blood cholesterol is a clear sign of a raised risk of heart attack and stroke, see pp. 82–3. It has been shown that in a minority, blood cholesterol increases when foods rich in cholesterol such as liver, eggs, and shellfish are eaten. However, in most people the cause of raised blood cholesterol levels is an unbalanced diet. The most effective way to reduce raised blood cholesterol levels is to eat less saturated fat, rather than avoiding high-cholesterol foods. In addition, stop smoking, lose weight if necessary, and get more exercise to help reduce raised cholesterol levels.

In recent years, a distinction has been drawn between "good" blood cholesterol, known as high density lipoprotein, or HDL, which is protective, and "bad" low density lipoprotein, or LDL, which encourages cholesterol to accumulate in the arteries, see pp. 82–3.

POLYUNSATURATED FATTY ACIDS

Two groups of polyunsaturated fatty acids (PUFAs) are known as omega-6 and omega-3 fatty acids, named after the number of double bonds in their chemical structure. The omega-6 linoleic fatty acid and the omega-3 alpha linolenic fatty acid are known as "essential" because we must obtain them from food: from these the body should be able to make up the other PUFAs.

The PUFAs have many functions in the body. Some of the omega-3 fatty acids are linked to a lower risk of fatal heart attack. These are

Sunflower seeds *are one of the best sources of omega-6 linoleic fatty acid, as well as vitamin E.*

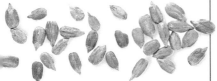

Oily fish and walnuts *Both supply omega-3 polyunsaturated fatty acids, which are linked to a reduced risk of fatal heart attack and also act against blood clots and inflammation.*

mainly found in oily fish, while linseed, walnuts, soybeans, purslane, and wheat germ provide the "parent" alpha-linolenic acid. Linoleic acid reduces blood cholesterol, and is plentiful in nuts, seeds, and the oils made from them. We need only small amounts of PUFAs, no more than 10% of our calories in total – ¾ oz (20g) for a person eating 1,800 calories a day. Most of us eat enough omega-6s, but too little omega-3s, especially the type found in oily fish.

MONOUNSATURATED FATS

Oils high in monounsaturated fatty acids, such as olive, canola, and sesame, have a place in the diet too. As most people already eat almost enough polyunsaturated fats, mono-unsaturated fats are preferable for replacing saturated fats in cooking.

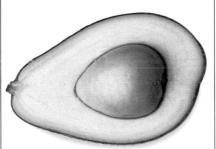

Avocado *The monounsaturated fat found in an avocado is healthier than saturated fat, but both types of fat are equally high in calories.*

Monounsaturated fats do not lower blood cholesterol levels as much as polyunsaturated fats, but they are better at maintaining levels of "good" HDL cholesterol. Unlike polyunsaturated fats, you can eat more of them without increasing your need for antioxidant vitamin E, and they can be heated to higher temperatures in cooking without oxidizing.

THE VITAMIN E FACTOR

The more polyunsaturated fats you eat, the more foods rich in vitamin E (and probably vitamin C) you need to eat.

All polyunsaturated fats are vulnerable to oxidation, a natural reaction with oxygen that in excess produces potentially harmful effects. In nature, foods high in polyunsaturated fats usually contain vitamin E, which protects against excess oxidation. But when foods are in storage much of this can be used up. Some vitamin E is also lost in processing; for example, whole-wheat bread has a significant amount, while white bread has only a trace. Oily fish and linseed are high in polyunsaturated fats but not in vitamin E, so it is wise to eat them with vitamin E-rich foods such as whole-wheat bread.

Favor foods that contain more vitamin E: a diet rich in this nutrient is emerging as one of the most protective factors against heart attack and degenerative diseases.

A HEALTHY BALANCE OF FATS

Eat more often

Foods rich in omega-3 polyunsaturated fatty acids such as oily fish, including salmon, mackerel, sardines, whitebait, herrings, and kippers; linseed; wheat germ; lower levels: walnuts; canola oil and soybeans.

Eat small amounts

Foods rich in omega-6 polyunsaturated fatty acids such as walnuts, sunflower seeds, and sunflower oil; wheat germ.

Eat less

Foods rich in saturated and trans fatty acids such as solid fats and dairy fats.

❖ PROTEIN ❖

PROTEIN-RICH FOODS

We need many types of protein for the structure and repair of cells, and to form hormones and enzymes. Our bodies make proteins by combining the basic components, about 20 amino acids. Adults must obtain 8 of these amino acids from food, and children must obtain 9. From these essential amino acids, our bodies can make the rest.

All 9 essential amino acids are present in any animal protein food, including eggs and milk, usually in a balance that suits our needs. This is not true of single plant protein foods, whether nuts, seeds, grains, or legumes, but a mixture of protein foods provides an ample supply.

Animal foods contain no fiber, and much dairy food and meat is very high in saturated fat. A key step in improving diet balance is to choose animal protein foods that are low in saturated fat, such as poultry, fish, game, lean meat, and low-fat milk and cheese, and eat them in only moderate amounts. Eating protein in the form of low-fat, high-fiber starchy foods and legumes lowers fat and raises fiber intake.

HOW MUCH PROTEIN DO YOU NEED?

It is recommended that 10–15% of the daily calorie intake should come from protein. The Western diet usually contains much more than this. Surplus protein is used as energy or stored, but excess protein unbalances the diet and can lead to calcium loss.

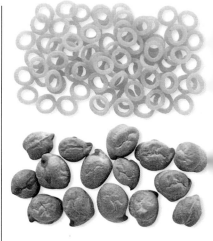

Complementary proteins *The amino acids in legumes, like beans, peas, and lentils, complement those in cereal grains, potatoes, or nuts. Pasta and chickpeas, for instance in a soup, are a good example of combining plant protein foods.*

❖ VITAMINS & MINERALS ❖

THE IMPORTANCE OF VITAMINS & MINERALS

There are about 15 vitamins and 15 minerals that are known to be needed in small amounts for human health and, except for vitamins D and K, they are available only from food. A lack of any of these micronutrients causes ill-health, either directly or by reducing resistance to disease.

In developed countries, nutrient shortage is mainly due to poor choice of food – for example, eating too little fresh fruit and vegetables, or too much alcohol or sugary or fatty foods – and to the loss of nutrients in food processing. Low-calorie diets also reduce nutrient intake. The less we eat, the more we need to choose food with a high level of nutrients per calorie. Foods vary in nutrient content, so eating a varied diet of high-nutrient foods is important to obtain each nutrient, and will supply most people's needs.

NUTRIENT SUPPLEMENTS

Vitamin and mineral supplements can be helpful – for example, for people who eat little – but they cannot make up for poor eating habits. Food provides a far more complex blend of nutrients and other substances. Increasing vitamin and mineral research can help us choose food that benefits us. It has also shown that, in some cases, massive amounts of a nutrient can be used as a medicinal drug, complete with potential side effects. But our growing knowledge emphasizes that we do not know enough about how our bodies use food to rely on supplements. Nutrients are part of an intricate balance, interacting with one another, varying in form and activity, and are affected by many other substances such as enzymes, acids, or fiber. Humans are adapted to eat a varied diet of food, not pills.

For a full listing of vitamins and minerals, their importance, function, and effects of shortage, see pp. 144–51.

Green leafy vegetables, *such as lettuce, are some of the most valuable foods, with a blend of vitamins, minerals, and other substances that no supplement could match.*

— ❖ SUBSTANCES WITH SPECIAL PROPERTIES ❖ —

THE ACTIVE CONSTITUENTS IN FOOD

Every food contains hundreds of substances besides the few that we know are valuable for providing energy or essential nutrients. These "non-nutrient" substances explain many of the effects of food, from the nose-clearing effect of chili peppers to the laxative effect of figs. Eating to improve health makes use of some of these special properties.

But it is not a simple case of one "active" ingredient being important, while the rest of the food is neutral. Very often a whole food turns out to have different effects from those of the known individual "active constituents."

Isolated substances do not share the safety record of the whole foodstuffs they come from. Furthermore, as with food in general, substances that are beneficial as part of a varied diet may be harmful in large, isolated amounts. It is safer to eat active constituents in a food form rather than in supplements.

Science now has better techniques to analyze the special properties of some foods and to give us the knowledge to use food to benefit our health. Research is in its early stages, and there can be no guarantees. But using foods in this way carries little risk either. The following are some of the compounds and active constituents that help to explain the health benefits of food.

ALLIUM COMPOUNDS

Onions and garlic contain several sulfur compounds that, during chopping or chewing, produce other compounds known to discourage blood clotting, and that in animal tests were shown to help increase cancer resistance. Chives and leeks contain much smaller

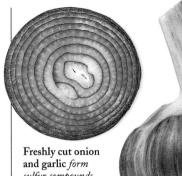

Freshly cut onion and garlic *form sulfur compounds that are one source of their health potential.*

amounts than onions and garlic. These useful compounds are volatile and easily dispersed, so it is not guaranteed that onion and garlic products contain them. As these active ingredients are linked to the smell of onion and garlic, any benefits may be reduced or lost with the smell, for example, after high-heat cooking.

ANTIOXIDANTS

Many substances in food can help the body's defenses in preventing the harmful effects from the by-products of oxidation. Oxidation occurs naturally in the human body when incomplete "free radical" oxygen molecules grab a hydrogen ion from a nearby molecule, which in turn grabs one from another structure, setting off a chain reaction that could lead to tissue damage. Without enough antioxidants, which prevent or stop the chain reaction, free radicals can multiply, putting stress on the body's defense systems. Free radicals in tobacco smoke and air pollutants add to the load.

It has been shown convincingly that those who eat more antioxidant-rich foods are less prone to heart disease, stroke, cataracts, and some cancers.

The major antioxidants from food that can help our defense system are vitamin E, several carotenes, and vitamin C. Many flavonoids, p. 22, have antioxidant properties, although it is not known how useful they are. In recent large-scale studies, supplements of beta-carotene and vitamin C showed no protective effect (although in some studies, supplements of vitamin E did), but eating foods rich in these antioxidants did have a protective effect. The evidence strongly suggests that it is best to eat antioxidants in foods, not supplements. Deficiency of selenium, zinc, or copper reduces antioxidant defenses, and excess iron can encourage oxidation.

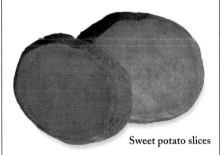

Sweet potato slices

Antioxidants in food *Red and orange vegetables and fruits are rich sources of antioxidant beta-carotene, with some vitamin C and E.*

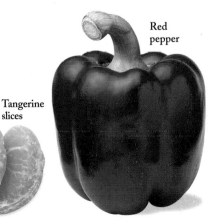

Red pepper

Tangerine slices

CAROTENES

Carotenes are the pigments that give most of the orange, red, and yellow color to vegetables and fruits. More than 500 carotenes have been identified, but until recently the only ones recognized as being important were alpha- and beta-carotene and cryptoxanthin because the body can convert these into vitamin A.

Carrots *The intense orange color of carrots reflects their high content of antioxidant carotenes.*

Now it is clear that these carotenes, as well as some others that have no link to vitamin A, have antioxidant properties. Since different carotenes vary in effect, it is sensible to eat a variety of them by eating a wide range of fruits and vegetables. In surveys, people who eat more foods rich in carotenes have a lower risk of heart disease, stroke, cataracts, and some forms of cancer, especially of the lung.

Beta-carotene taken in supplements has shown little or no benefit in tests, and researchers agree that the message is to eat carotenes in foods, not supplements.

Pumpkin and spinach *Leafy, dark green vegetables such as spinach are as high in carotenes as orange vegetables, but the color is masked by green chlorophyll.*

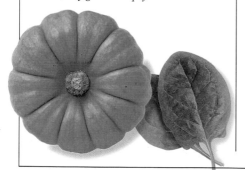

DIGESTIVE STIMULANTS

Perhaps we have an instinctive awareness that bitter-tasting substances stimulate the digestive system, because we choose many bitter-flavored drinks as apéritifs, for example, tonic water and vermouth.

Bitter flavors help the digestive system by stimulating its secretion of digestive juices. This in turn can improve digestion and the absorption of nutrients. Foods with a mild "bitter" note include artichokes and some salad greens, such as radicchio and Belgian endive.

Other, nonbitter, digestive stimulants include chili peppers, ginger, mustard oil plants such as watercress, and horseradish, fennel, celery, parsley, and cabbage and other cruciferous vegetables.

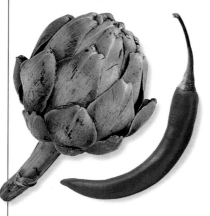

Artichoke and chili pepper *Foods that can help digestion include warming, digestive juice stimulants such as chili peppers, and artichokes, which encourage bile production.*

FLAVONOIDS

Nearly all fruits and vegetables contain some of the 4,000-plus flavonoids or polyphenols. The name "flavonoid" comes from the Latin *flavus*, or yellow, the color of many of these varied substances.

The main flavonoid groups are flavones, flavonols, catechins, tannins, isoflavones (the main phytoestrogens in soybeans, see

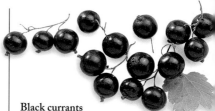

Black currants *Anthocyanin flavonoids are the pigments that give purple, blue, and deep red colors to fruit such as black currants, blueberries, and black cherries.*

p. 23), and anthocyanins. A single food is likely to contain a range of these flavonoids. For example, 40 flavonoids have been isolated from citrus fruits alone.

In the laboratory, individual flavonoids have displayed a wide variety of actions: antioxidant, anti-inflammatory, antiviral or antibacterial, and sometimes more than one of these. We still understand little about how flavonoids work in the body, or how much is absorbed from different kinds of food. Varying laboratory tests showed that the common flavonoid quercetin, for example, can either benefit or harm cells. Yet in Dutch and Finnish studies, people who usually ate more quercetin, for instance in onions, had lower rates of heart disease and stroke in later years.

Recent studies suggest that flavonoids are promising health protectors, probably due to circulation benefits and antioxidant effects. Onions are especially high in quercetin, followed by tea, red wine, and apples.

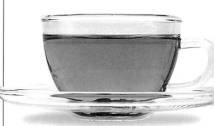

Tea *Tannin flavonoids give the tongue-tightening tingle to tea; drinking tea with milk does not affect its flavonoid availability.*

FRIENDLY MICROFLORA

We are all familiar with antibiotics, the medicines that kill bacteria. Now there is growing research interest in "probiotics": substances that can provide more of the live, intestinal microflora – "friendly" bacteria that are present naturally in the gut and are a key part of resistance to illness.

There are hundreds of types of safe bacteria: research is under way to identify those with health benefits. For years, medical opinion held that friendly microflora in food would not reach the intestines alive due to stomach acids. But research confirms that some bacteria do survive digestion, and that probiotics can be useful, especially for diarrhea and loss of disease resistance after food poisoning or taking antibiotics.

Bacteria that have shown health benefits are mainly varieties of *Lactobacillus acidophilus*, *Bulgaricus*, and *Bifidobacteria* found in types of yogurt, or in raw sauerkraut.

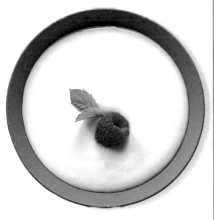

Live yogurt *Only yogurt that has not been heat-treated or pasteurized contains active microflora cultures, which give it special properties.*

"Prebiotics" is a new term for foods that can encourage the friendly bacteria we already have. Prebiotic foods contain carbohydrates that resist digestion by the body. The most notable prebiotic foods are artichokes, endive, and linseed.

GLUCOSINOLATES

These sulfur compounds are found in cabbage, broccoli, and other cruciferous vegetables.

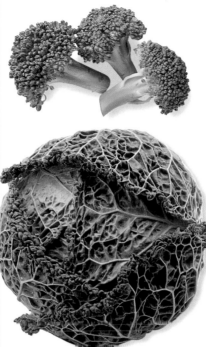

Broccoli and cabbage *Brassica varieties of cruciferous vegetables such as broccoli, cabbage, and Brussels sprouts are high in glucosinolates.*

When the cell walls of these vegetables are broken by cutting or chewing, compounds called isothiocyanates and indoles are formed. In several animal trials and one human trial, these have been found to discourage cancer, while in many population studies, people who eat more of these vegetables show lower rates of several cancers.

More of these isothiocyanates and indoles compounds are formed when there is plenty of vitamin C present, so it is important not to overcook vegetables rich in glucosinolates. Different cruciferous vegetables produce different kinds and amounts of isothiocyanates and indoles. It is not yet known how they work or the most beneficial sources.

PHYTOESTROGENS

Many seeds, grains, vegetables, and fruits contain a range of naturally occurring chemicals that are similar enough in structure to the female hormone estrogen to mimic its activity in the body. Foods with substantial levels of phytoestrogens include soybeans, linseed, fennel, whole wheat, and legumes.

It is not yet possible to measure the estrogenlike effects of phytoestrogens, but all are much weaker than a woman's own estrogen, or than that used in oral contraceptives or hormone-replacement therapy.

Because excess estrogen is linked to infertility and a higher risk of breast cancer, there is some concern over the activity of phytoestrogens in food. Yet in countries such as Japan, where women eat more soybeans, one of the foods highest in phytoestrogens, far fewer women develop breast cancer. Researchers are now testing the theory that, in younger women, weak estrogenic compounds from food may be of benefit by supplanting stronger estrogen, lowering levels in the body, see p. 87. Research suggests that postmenopausal women may benefit from the estrogenic effect provided by phytoestrogen-rich foods, see p. 87.

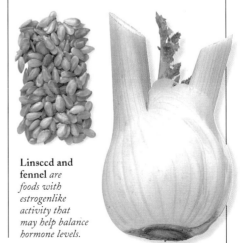

Linseed and fennel *are foods with estrogenlike activity that may help balance hormone levels.*

DIGESTION & ABSORPTION

OUR SUPPLY OF NUTRIENTS depends on not only what foods we eat, but how well we digest and absorb them. We do not extract all the vitamins or minerals present in food, and official recommended intakes of nutrients allow for this. Absorbing small amounts of vitamins or minerals is not always bad: the body may not require all the nutrients supplied and may use low absorption to protect itself from excess. Sometimes, however, for various reasons the digestive system is unable to extract or absorb the nutrients it needs. To ensure a good supply of nutrients, the digestive system has to break down food efficiently into molecules that can be absorbed through the wall of the digestive tract. Its other task, equally vital to our health, is to dispose of unwanted substances from food and body processes.

❖ THE DIGESTIVE SYSTEM ❖

BREAKING DOWN FOOD INTO NUTRIENTS

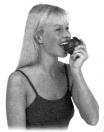

1 *The teeth crush food into small pieces, which will make it easier for enzymes in the stomach to make contact with each food molecule. Enzymes in saliva begin to break down starch before the food passes through the esophagus into the stomach.*

2 *In the stomach, digestive enzymes (produced in response to chewing and the smell of food) begin to break down protein. Hydrochloric acid in the stomach destroys most bacteria in food and water. Muscular contractions in the stomach churn the food into a semi-liquid consistency, after which it passes into the duodenum, the first part of the small intestine.*

3 *The liver produces bile, which is stored in the gallbladder and then released into the duodenum. Bile emulsifies fats into tiny droplets. The pancreas also releases digestive juices into the duodenum. These contain enzymes that break carbohydrates, proteins, and fats down more.*

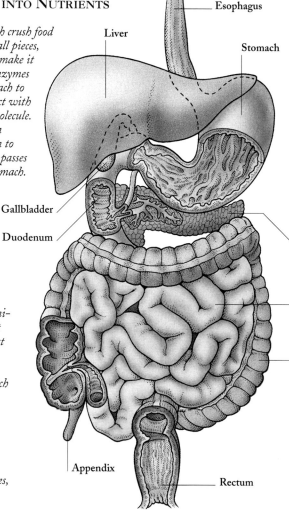

Esophagus

Liver

Stomach

Gallbladder

Duodenum

Pancreas

Small intestine

Large intestine (colon)

Appendix

Rectum

4 *Some nutrients go straight into the bloodstream through the stomach wall, but most are absorbed from the small intestine, which has a huge surface area to facilitate the absorption of nutrients. Its wall is covered with countless tiny fronds called villi.*

As the molecules of nutrients pass through the small intestine, they are absorbed into the lining and then pass directly into the bloodstream, from where they are distributed to cells to be used or, in some cases, stored in the body as needed.

5 *Finally, water and the unwanted parts of food pass into the large intestine. Here, much of the water is absorbed back into the body through the lining of the colon. Undigested matter and other body wastes are then expelled as feces.*

❖ NUTRIENT ABSORPTION ❖

FACTORS THAT REDUCE NUTRIENT ABSORPTION

Any illness that impedes digestion reduces nutrient absorption, for example, liver disorders that prevent bile production, and Crohn's disease or diarrhea. Alcohol abuse, which damages the liver, is also a common cause of reduced nutrient absorption. Many medicines such as strong laxatives, aluminum antacids, diuretics, and some steroids reduce the absorption of nutrients, especially vitamins A, B_6, D, E, K, and folic acid.

Poor nutrient absorption can also be due to an allergy. People with lactose intolerance, for example, are unable to digest milk. For people with celiac disease, the gluten protein found in wheat, rye, and barley destroys or flattens the villi in the small intestine, which hinders the absorption of many nutrients.

In older people, smaller amounts of digestive juices are produced in the stomach and pancreas, reducing the uptake of iron, calcium, folic acid, and vitamin B_{12}.

Although high-fiber foods are rich in minerals, they should not be eaten in excess. Fiber limits the overall absorption of iron, calcium, and zinc from other foods eaten at the same meal, especially if the fiber is high in phytic acid. Wheat bran and oat bran are very high in phytic acid. This is reduced during breadmaking, however, so eating whole-wheat bread is the best way to eat bran.

Tea contains tannins, which sharply cut the absorption of iron from food eaten at the same time. Drinking strong tea regularly with meals encourages anemia.

If you are taking long-term medication or suffer from ulcerative colitis or bouts of diarrhea, seek advice on diet and a possible need for supplements.

HOW TO IMPROVE NUTRIENT ABSORPTION

Helping our digestive system absorb the nutrients we need starts with our eating habits. Individuals vary widely in what their digestive system can cope with, but anything that regularly causes discomfort is also likely to reduce nutrient absorption.

Digestive juices flow more freely if we eat only when hungry, relaxed, and attracted by the look and smell of food. Do not assume that indigestion is due to excess acid and take antacids: look at your eating habits first, and choose more foods that help digestion, such as artichokes, chili peppers, fennel, watercress, celery, parsley, and bitter salad greens – for example, radicchio and Belgian endive.

High-fat foods are a common cause of sluggish digestion. They make the digestive system work harder because fat must be broken down into tiny droplets.

Eating plenty of foods rich in insoluble fiber and digestion-resistant starch, such as starchy foods and whole-wheat bread, shortens the transit time of food and body wastes, and so reduces our exposure to possibly harmful substances.

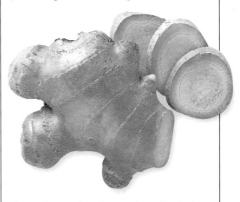

Digestive stimulants, *such as ginger, aid digestion by increasing the flow of digestive juices. Ginger is also warming and eases colic.*

Iron absorption from plant foods is improved by eating vitamin C-rich foods and avoiding large amounts of calcium at the same meal. Zinc and iron from plant and dairy foods are better absorbed if some meat or fish protein is also in the meal. Calcium absorption is best stimulated by weight-bearing exercise and needs adequate vitamin D supplied by sunlight on the skin or by oily fish. Do not take antibiotics unnecessarily as they damage "friendly" microflora, which produce some B vitamins and vitamin K.

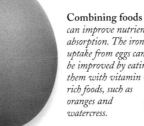

Combining foods *can improve nutrient absorption. The iron uptake from eggs can be improved by eating them with vitamin C–rich foods, such as oranges and watercress.*

SPECIAL DIETARY NEEDS

AS WE GROW OLDER our nutrient needs change. We expect teenage boys, for example, to eat us "out of house and home," but we attribute this habit to their increasing energy requirements, rather than to a rising need for nutrients. In many cases, we unconsciously adjust to changes in nutrient requirements. Most people approaching middle age gradually eat less, but it may take a long time before they look back and realize how much their eating patterns have changed. Sometimes we do not adapt our eating habits instinctively: for example, people gain excess weight if they do not reduce their calorie intake to suit lower energy use; and teenagers often use up a large number of calories on soft drinks rather than on foods which would provide them with more nutrients. As our nutrient needs change during particular stages of life, certain foods and eating habits can help us to adjust more effectively.

❖ PUBERTY ❖

NUTRIENT NEEDS

Healthy eating is rarely a priority for young people, yet the growth spurt of children in the adolescent years causes a jump in their requirement for most nutrients. This is especially true of calcium and iron, which young people need more of than adults because they are using these minerals for rapidly forming extra bone and tissue.

Lack of calcium can affect bone growth, which peaks during the the mid-teen years. The bone strength laid down at this time can affect the risk of osteoporosis in middle age.

Girls often restrict their food intake because they want to be thin, just as puberty is making them curvier. Their iron requirement roughly doubles at puberty as extra needs for growth coincide with the loss of iron during menstruation. Up to a quarter of teenage girls are likely to be iron-deficient, affecting their energy levels, resistance to infection, and, in some cases, academic performance. Many teenage girls become vegetarian and need to take extra care to eat iron-rich foods.

Vegetarian leanings often overlap with a desire to control weight, and may mask the development of eating disorders such as anorexia. Zinc deficiency, which reduces taste and appetite, is thought to play a part in some cases. Boys are increasingly affected by the fashion for thin bodies, with similar risks to their health.

The level of sugar eaten by many older children is very high. This increases tooth decay and reduces their chances of obtaining a balanced diet. Teaching young people how to put together a balanced diet is important so that they can obtain the nutrients they need without following so many of their parents in becoming overweight. Lack of variety is often a feature of teenage eating habits, and introducing younger children to as wide a range of foods as possible, especially fresh vegetables and fruits, helps guard against this.

SPECIAL VALUE FOODS

Eat more often
....
• Calcium-rich foods: yogurt, hard cheese, milk, tofu, almonds, green leafy vegetables, sardines
• Iron-rich foods: chicken liver, dried apricots, legumes, red meat, oily fish, green leafy vegetables
• Zinc-rich foods: shellfish, lean meat, pumpkin seeds

Avoid
....
• Large amounts of sugar are not desirable even for very active teenagers
• Wheat bran, except in whole-wheat bread

❖ PREGNANCY ❖

SPECIAL VALUE FOODS

Eat more often

• Calcium-rich foods: yogurt, almonds, tofu, salad greens, sardines, whitebait
• Fiber-rich foods: dried apricots, linseed
• Folic acid- and iron-rich foods: red meat, cruciferous vegetables, watercress, wheat germ, legumes
• Omega-3-rich oily fish, linseed

Avoid

• Pregnant women are advised not to eat liver. Excess retinol vitamin A (but not beta-carotene) can cause fetal abnormalities
• Food poisoning carries extra risks

NUTRIENT NEEDS

It is important to eat well for several months before conceiving to build up your nutritional status. Critical developments in fetal nerve and brain development take place in the first 3–4 weeks, a period when most women do not yet know that they are pregnant. Folic acid reduces the risk of neural tube defects and women planning to conceive should take 400mcg folic acid a day until they are 12 weeks pregnant, and eat foods rich in folic acid during their pregnancy.

If you are planning a pregnancy, avoid being underweight and give up smoking and alcohol. This helps guard against having a low birthweight or premature baby, who has a far higher risk of poor health.

During pregnancy, it is more important to improve the quality of your diet than to eat more. Although iron needs rise, it is better to eat iron-rich foods than it is to take supplements, unless hemoglobin levels are low. Many mothers eat little omega-3 fatty acids, critical for fetal brain development.

❖ OLDER PEOPLE ❖

NUTRIENT NEEDS

As we get older, we need fewer calories but similar amounts of nutrients, so it becomes even more important to choose foods that provide higher levels of nutrients per calorie. The drop in caloric needs is due to a slower metabolism, and in most people, less activity.

Keeping active allows you to eat more food and nutrients without becoming overweight, which increases the risk of joint problems, diabetes, gallstones, and other illnesses. Keeping active also

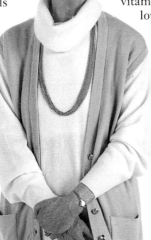

helps prevent depression, poor circulation, and excess bone loss.

In many older people, nutrient absorption declines. Levels of zinc and vitamins B6 and D are often low, reducing the body's immunity and general well-being.

In the elderly, especially the less active, improving nutrition has shown dramatic benefits, for instance, cutting down the hospital recovery time after surgery, reducing infections, and in some cases helping reduce mental confusion.

SPECIAL VALUE FOODS

Eat more often

• Antioxidant-rich foods, see p. 21
• Digestive stimulants to help absorption: chili peppers, artichokes, watercress
• Zinc-rich foods for the immune system: shellfish, pumpkin seeds, chicken liver
• Fiber-rich foods: whole-wheat bread, linseed, sunflower seeds
• Oily fish to provide vitamin D and essential fatty acids
• Potassium-rich fruit and juice

Avoid

• Wheat bran, except in whole-wheat bread
• Dehydration: drink ample fluid

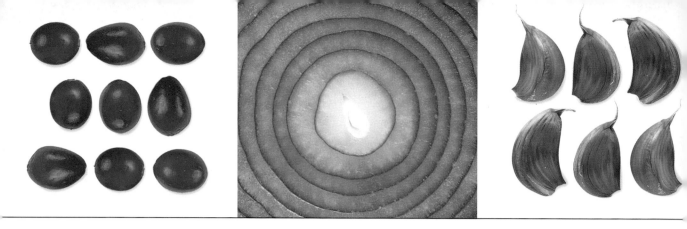

50 FOOD PROFILES

A photographic catalog of 50 key foods with outstanding benefits,

supported by scientific and traditional evidence. Choosing these delicious foods

more often is one of the most effective ways to safeguard your health.

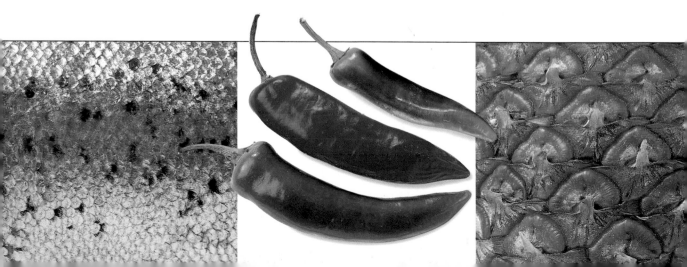

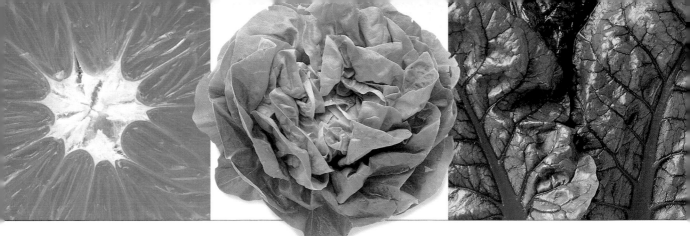

BONUS FOODS

Twenty popular foods with star ability to help your health.
These foods combine exceptional nutritional value with the bonus
of special properties that can help combat many common
and major diseases. Profiles of each food give details of nutritional
value, therapeutic use, and how much to eat, while culinary
know-how reveals how to tap into their benefits.

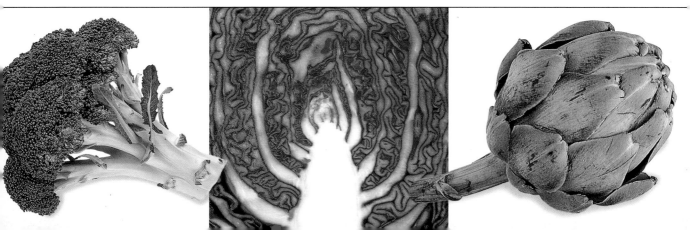

HEALTH BENEFITS

Assists liver function

Aids digestion and helps gallbladder problems

Can lower cholesterol levels

Can reduce fluid retention

May help stabilize blood sugar levels

ARTICHOKE

DELICIOUS AND ELEGANT, globe artichokes have been eaten as a vegetable since Roman times and known as an aid to digestion since the 16th century. Artichokes are helpful for the gallbladder, liver, and kidneys. Despite their shared name, Jerusalem artichokes are not botanically related.

KEY NUTRITIONAL VALUES

per 9oz (250g) cooked large globe artichoke, weighed whole

Calories (kcal)	20
Folic acid (mcg)	50
Iron (mg)	0.5
Niacin (mg)	1
Potassium (mg)	330
Zinc (mg)	0.5

❖ HEALTH & NUTRITION ❖

THERAPEUTIC PROPERTIES

• *Protects and supports liver and bile health*
Artichokes are traditionally used in European pharmaceutical remedies to help the liver, the gallbladder, and digestion. Like other "bitter" vegetables, artichokes increase bile output, and in studies they relieved liver-related gallbladder or abdominal discomfort.

• *Can reduce fat and cholesterol levels*
In German studies (1975, 1980), artichoke extract substantially lowered volunteers' blood fats and cholesterol. The reduction that can be achieved by eating artichoke itself has not yet been quantified.

• *Traditional diuretic*
Eating artichokes increases the flow of urine and can help relieve fluid retention.

• *Helpful for diabetics*
Traditionally, artichokes have been recommended for diabetics. They contain inulin, a form of starch that resists digestion, and may limit the rise in blood sugar levels after eating.

Color ranges from pale gold to lavender

HOW MUCH TO EAT
Eat large or small, lightly cooked artichokes freely. Bottled or canned baby artichokes and artichoke hearts are a useful alternative to fresh.

Globe artichokes *belong to the thistle family and grow easily in temperate gardens.*

Hairy "choke"

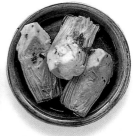

Artichoke hearts *are bottled or canned for use in the winter months.*

❖ IN THE KITCHEN ❖

CHOOSING & STORING
Large varieties are best for eating leaf-by-leaf and for making prepared hearts. Look for tender green heads without brown patches. The hairy "choke" between the head and leaves must be removed from large artichokes before eating. Artichokes toughen with storage. Store them, wrapped, in the refrigerator to slow moisture loss.

COOKING & EATING
Small artichoke heads can be eaten whole, cooked, and very thinly sliced, with an oil dressing, or sautéed and added to dishes such as risotto. To cook a large artichoke, simmer it in unsalted water for 35–40 minutes until a leaf comes away from the base easily. Artichoke leaves are eaten hot or cold, often dipped in a sauce.

RECIPES
Artichoke Heart Salad 109
Artichoke Frittata 120

BROCCOLI

TENDER, BUTTERY-TASTING broccoli shines out of many research studies as a food with health-building and cancer-preventing potential. Like other members of the cabbage family, broccoli contains particular chemicals that are known to discourage cancer, and is also rich in a range of nutrients.

HEALTH BENEFITS

Can reduce risk of cancer

♦

Helps lower risk of heart disease and stroke

♦

May reduce risk of cataracts

♦

Lessens risk of spina bifida

♦

Helps to combat anemia

♦

Rich in nutrients

KEY NUTRITIONAL VALUES

per ¼ lb (100g) raw green broccoli

Calories (kcal)	33
Beta-carotene (mcg)	575
Calcium (mg)	56
Folic acid (mcg)	90
Iron (mg)	1.7
Vitamin C (mg)	87
Vitamin E (mg)	1.3
Zinc (mg)	0.6

❖ HEALTH & NUTRITION ❖

THERAPEUTIC PROPERTIES

• *Guards against cancer*
American studies (1977–78) revealed that people who ate broccoli daily had a lower risk of lung cancer. Other studies have shown that people who eat more cruciferous vegetables, such as broccoli, have lower rates of cancer, especially cancer of the colon.

• *High in the antioxidants beta-carotene and vitamins C and E*
Large-scale surveys have shown that people with high antioxidant levels in the body from food, rather than from supplements, have a lower risk of heart disease, stroke, cataracts, and cancer.

• *Rich source of folic acid and iron*
Broccoli, especially purple sprouting broccoli, is an excellent source of folic acid, which women planning a pregnancy need plenty of to reduce the risk of having a baby with spina bifida. Iron and folic acid help prevent or correct anemia.

• *Exceptionally rich in vitamins and minerals*
Broccoli combines high levels of folic acid, antioxidants, B vitamins, calcium, iron, and zinc. It is a great vegetable.

Purple sprouting broccoli

HOW MUCH TO EAT
Purple sprouting and green broccoli contain more calcium and folic acid than other varieties. About 1–3 6oz (170g) servings of broccoli a week are likely to lower the risk of cancer. For women planning a pregnancy, a 6oz (170g) serving of purple sprouting broccoli, cooked lightly in little or no water, provides over half of the recommended daily intake of folic acid.

Head of green broccoli

·········· *Important note* ··········
Broccoli reduces iodine absorption. People who eat broccoli more than 2–3 times a week should ensure that they eat iodine-rich foods, especially if they live in an area with low soil iodine.

❖ IN THE KITCHEN ❖

CHOOSING & STORING
The stalks and leaves of sprouting forms have similar properties to the florets. Look for organically grown broccoli. Select firm spears, avoiding woody, browning, or yellowing stalks, which are a sign of toughening, bitter tops. Store broccoli, wrapped, in the warmest part of the refrigerator and use as quickly as possible.

COOKING & EATING
Freshly cut broccoli is sweet and tender enough to be eaten raw in salads, and the small florets are delicious with mayonnaise or dips. To cook broccoli, steam or boil it briefly in very little water, with a tight-fitting lid, until just tender. Lightly cooked broccoli has a delicate taste that complements a wide variety of foods.

RECIPES
Vegetable Chowder 103
Arame, Broccoli & Walnut Salad 110
Broccoli Stir-Fry 121

CABBAGE

IN RESEARCH CABBAGE stands out for its health value. Dozens of studies show that cabbage and other cruciferous vegetables are protective foods. All are good sources of vitamins, minerals, and fiber and now it is known that they can help in other ways too. Cabbage can be enjoyed in many recipes.

HEALTH BENEFITS

Can reduce risk of cancer

Helps lower risk of heart disease and stroke

May cut risk of cataracts

Speeds ulcer healing and improves digestive health

Helps cut risk of spina bifida

KEY NUTRITIONAL VALUES

per ¼ lb (100g) raw cabbage

Calories (kcal)	26
B vitamins	Good source
Beta-carotene (mcg)	385
Calcium (mg)	52
Folic acid (mcg)	75
Potassium (mg)	270
Vitamin C (mg)	50
Vitamin E (mg)	0.2

❖ HEALTH & NUTRITION ❖

THERAPEUTIC PROPERTIES

• *Contains antioxidants and other substances that improve disease resistance*
In population surveys, people who eat cabbage often have a lower rate of cancer, especially of the stomach, colon, lung, and skin. People with high levels of antioxidants in the body from food also have lower rates of heart disease, stroke, and cataracts.

• *Helps peptic ulcers*
The efficacy of raw cabbage juice as a traditional ulcer remedy is supported by tests on volunteers. Raw cabbage is also helpful, but has a weaker effect.

• *Raw sauerkraut contains micro-organisms good for intestinal flora*
Sauerkraut (fermented cabbage) is traditionally used to improve digestion and gut health.

• *Raw green cabbage is a rich source of folic acid*
Ample folic acid lowers the risk of having a baby with spina bifida.

HOW MUCH TO EAT
Even 1 serving of cabbage a week, either raw, cooked, or as sauerkraut, may lower the risk of colon cancer. Studies suggest that for a general protective effect, 2–3 helpings a week are needed. Raw green cabbage contains the most folic acid and antioxidants.

..... ***Important note*** .....
As cabbage reduces iodine absorption, people who eat cabbage more than 2–3 times a week should ensure they eat iodine-rich foods, especially if they live in an area with low soil iodine.

Savoy cabbage

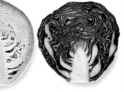

Green cabbage   Red cabbage

❖ IN THE KITCHEN ❖

CHOOSING & STORING
Choose the freshest cabbage and use it quickly, before it toughens. If using the outer leaves, look for organic varieties to avoid farm chemical residues. Store, wrapped, in the refrigerator. Only raw sauerkraut contains "live" bacteria (which survive freezing). Sauerkraut that is heat-treated for canning or bottling has little or no bacteria.

COOKING & EATING
Whether braised, stuffed, added to soups or stir-fries, or eaten raw in slaw salads, there is such a variety of cabbage recipes that everyone, even the least enthusiastic cabbage-eater, should be able to find some they like. To help reduce flatulence, combine cabbage with a carminative spice or herb, such as caraway or fennel seeds.

RECIPES
Slaw Salad 112
Oden-Style Stuffed Cabbage 122
Braised Red Cabbage 126

CARROT

CARROTS ARE NOT ONLY good for you, they are also excellent value. The orange color of carrots comes from the carotenes, see p. 22. These were once thought to be useful only for the body to convert into vitamin A. Today, foods rich in carotenes are known to have many other health benefits.

HEALTH BENEFITS

Helps protect against cancer, especially lung cancer

◆

Can lower blood cholesterol

◆

Helps guard against food poisoning

KEY NUTRITIONAL VALUES

per ¼ lb (100g) raw carrot

Calories (kcal)	30
Carotenes, including beta-carotene (mcg)	8,115
Fiber (g)	2.4
Vitamin C (mg)	6
Vitamin E (mg)	0.6

❖ HEALTH & NUTRITION ❖

THERAPEUTIC PROPERTIES

• *Can reduce risk of lung cancer*
Studies have shown that people who eat carrots regularly, including smokers, are far less likely to suffer lung cancer. This has been linked to the high level of beta-carotene in carrots. Beta-carotene from pills does not show the same results, suggesting that carrots have other protective factors not yet recognized.

• *Helps guard against other forms of cancer*
In studies of large groups of people, a high beta-carotene intake from carrots and other vegetables and fruits is linked with up to 50% lower rates of cancer of the bladder, cervix, colon, prostate, larynx, and esophagus, and a 20% reduction in the risk of postmenopausal breast cancer.

• *A simple way to lower blood cholesterol*
In 1979, a Scottish trial showed that healthy volunteers eating 7oz (200g) raw carrots a day for 3 weeks reduced their blood cholesterol levels by 11%. Levels rose when they stopped.

• *Helps prevent food poisoning*
Trials have shown that even small amounts of raw carrot can kill listeria and other food-poisoning organisms.

Unless organically grown, carrots should be peeled

Orange color comes from carotenes

HOW MUCH TO EAT
Eat freely. Carrots are the richest common source of beta-carotene, so eating just 1 large carrot a day increases the level of beta-carotene in the body.

Fresh carrots *have more beneficial properties than carrot juice.*

❖ IN THE KITCHEN ❖

CHOOSING & STORING
Carrots are particularly prone to high pesticide and other farm chemical residues and should always be peeled before use, unless organically grown. Older carrots contain higher amounts of beta-carotene than spring carrots. To keep carrots crisp, store them in the vegetable drawer of the refrigerator or in a cool place.

COOKING & EATING
Carrots add color as well as crunch and flavor to many dishes. Varieties range from the super-sweet, especially spring carrots, to the fuller flavor of the fall crop. Beta-carotene is not destroyed by cooking. Raw carrots can be finely or coarsely grated, cut into matchsticks or fingers and served with dips, or added to soups.

RECIPES
Carrot & Cilantro Soup 100
Slaw Salad 112
Beef & Carrot Tzimmes 118
Polish Carrot Cake 135

LETTUCE & SALAD GREENS

THERE ARE MORE THAN one hundred types of lettuces and salad greens. Although often dismissed as being mostly water, leafy salad greens contain valuable amounts of vitamins, minerals, and antioxidants. They also have an important advantage, when compared to other foods, in that they are nearly always eaten raw.

HEALTH BENEFITS

Help reduce risk of cancer

◆

Can reduce risk of heart disease, stroke, and cataracts

◆

Help prevent spina bifida and anemia

◆

Aid digestion and liver health

◆

May ease nervous insomnia

KEY NUTRITIONAL VALUES

per ¼ lb (100g) lettuce and salad greens, average amounts

Calories (kcal)	14
Carotenes (mcg)	355
Folic acid (mcg)	55
Iron (mg)	0.7
Potassium (mg)	220
Vitamin C (mg)	5
Vitamin E (mg)	0.57

❖ HEALTH & NUTRITION ❖

THERAPEUTIC PROPERTIES

• *Guard against cancer*
Nineteen population studies have linked eating lettuce and salad greens frequently with a lower risk of cancer, especially of the stomach.

• *Combine the antioxidants vitamins C and E and carotenes*
Levels of carotenes and vitamin C are much higher in the green, outer leaves of lettuce than the pale inner leaves, carotenes by as much as 50 times. A higher intake of foods rich in antioxidants is linked to lower rates of cancer, heart disease, stroke, and cataracts.

• *Good source of folic acid and iron*
Folic acid and iron help prevent and treat anemia. For women planning a pregnancy, folic acid reduces the risk of having a baby with spina bifida. Pale iceberg lettuce has as high a level of folic acid as green lettuce. Endive and chard are also very rich sources. Endive is the richest source of iron with 2.8mg per 3½ oz (100g) serving; Boston lettuce is a good source, with 1.5mg per 3½ oz (100g).

• *Traditional digestive and liver stimulant*
Radicchio, Belgian endive, curly endive, escarole, and other bitter salad greens stimulate digestive fluids and liver function, which in traditional medicine is believed to help gout and rheumatism.

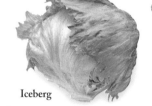

Green outer leaves contain the most antioxidants

Iceberg

Romaine

Boston

❖ IN THE KITCHEN ❖

CHOOSING & STORING
To obtain the highest level of nutrients, look for untrimmed lettuce and salad greens with the most green, outer leaves. Salad leaves should be as fresh and crisp as possible. Prewashed, packaged salads with torn leaves lose their vitamin C and folic acid content quickly. Store lettuce and salad greens in the refrigerator, wrapped and covered, to protect them from light and heat, and use as quickly as possible.

PREPARING & EATING
Fresh salads are best prepared as closely as possible to the time when they will be eaten. Exposure of cut surfaces to air quickly diminishes both the eating quality and nutritional value of lettuce and salad greens. Thoroughly washing the leaves removes not only chemical residues, but also infectious agents such as listeria. Leaves should be torn rather than cut, and dried if the salad dressing is to coat them well.

RECIPES
Green Shchi Soup 102
Artichoke Heart Salad 109
Sunflower Green
Salad 112
Honey & Mustard
Dressing 140
Yogurt & Mint
Dressing 141

• *Sedative effect*
The white "milk" that seeps out of a cut lettuce base has been used to calm the nerves and promote sleep since Roman times. There is less milk in modern cultivated lettuce, but many people still find it soporific.

• *Purslane provides essential fatty acids*
Purslane has an extraordinarily high level of omega-3 essential fatty acids, comparable to the levels provided by oily fish. Early herbalists praised it as a cooling medicine, good for gout and other "hot" aches, and headaches. The anti-inflammatory effects of omega-3 fatty acids, now confirmed by research, suggest these uses are justified.

• *Sorrel is a traditional diuretic*
Sorrel is traditionally used, in small amounts, to increase urine production; for example, to relieve fluid retention.

HOW MUCH TO EAT
Eat leafy salad greens freely, organically grown if possible, as the leaves have a large surface area exposed to pesticides. A generous salad that includes chard and endive easily provides almost half the amount of folic acid advised for women planning a pregnancy.
If you eat large amounts of salad with oil dressings, consider lower-fat dressings.

.... ***Important note*** ....
People with gout, kidney stones, or rheumatism should avoid sorrel because it is rich in oxalates.

Red-stemmed chard

Sorrel

Escarole

Curly endive

ONION

IT IS GOOD TO KNOW THAT a food most of us already eat often can do so much for our health. As some of the health benefits of onions are linked to their volatile smell, which is released when fresh onions are cut, it is best to keep cooking with plenty of fresh onions instead of commerical onion products.

HEALTH BENEFITS

Helps reduce risk of heart disease and stroke

Natural antibiotic action

Relieves congestion in airways

Can help bronchial congestion

Aids cancer resistance

KEY NUTRITIONAL VALUES

per ¼ lb (100g) raw onion, peeled weight

Calories (kcal)	36
B vitamins	Wide range
Fiber (g)	1.4
Niacin (mg)	0.7
Potassium (mg)	160

❖ HEALTH & NUTRITION ❖

THERAPEUTIC PROPERTIES

• *Counters the rise in cholesterol and blood clotting after a fatty meal*
In most people, blood cholesterol levels and the tendency to form blood clots rise after eating a high-fat meal, but not if the meal includes onion, raw or cooked.

• *Helps reduce total cholesterol and high blood pressure, and to raise levels of "good" cholesterol*
People who regularly eat raw onions have healthier levels of blood fats. In a 1985 study, onion reduced high blood pressure in 13 out of 20 sufferers, and high blood cholesterol in 9 out of 18 volunteers with high levels.

• *Helps combat infections*
Onions are a traditional remedy for infectious illnesses, such as colds, coughs, bronchitis, and gastric infections.

• *Counters bronchial constriction*
There is some scientific research to support the traditional use of freshly cut onions to prevent asthma.

• *Helps cancer resistance*
Frequent onion eaters have less cancer risk, perhaps due to the allium compounds and flavonoids in onions, see pp. 21–22.

Raw onion is more likely than cooked onion to raise "good" cholesterol levels

Yellow onion

Red onion

Scallions *have a health advantage because they are usually eaten raw.*

Shallots

HOW MUCH TO EAT
Freshly cut raw onions have the widest and most reliable health benefits, but cooked onions help too. Trials suggest that regularly eating 2oz (60g) raw or cooked onion with a meal, or about half an onion a day, has good effects on health.

❖ IN THE KITCHEN ❖

CHOOSING & STORING
Many people find that sweeter, milder onion varieties are more appealing for eating raw. Store onions in the vegetable drawer of the refrigerator, avoiding dampness, or in a cool place. Onion products, such as dried onion, where the smell is reduced, are unlikely to be as beneficial.

COOKING & EATING
Only those who have had to cook without onions fully appreciate their value. You can make more of onions by increasing their amount in recipes, and using traditional recipes, such as roast onions. To retain the maximum amount of valuable substances, cut onions close to serving or cooking time.

RECIPES
Swiss Onion Soup 102
Onions à la Grecque 107
Munkazina Salad 109
Roast Onions 126

SWEET POTATO

LIKE CARROTS, ORANGE-FLESHED sweet potatoes are both savory and sweet. With far more vitamins than the unrelated ordinary potato, sweet potatoes combine valuable antioxidants and minerals. They are the only low-fat food with a high vitamin E level, rivaling rich sources such as nuts and seeds.

KEY NUTRITIONAL VALUES

per ¼ lb (100g) baked sweet potato

Calories (kcal)	115
Carotenes (mcg)	5,140
Fiber (g)	3.3
Iron (mg)	0.9
Potassium (mg)	480
Vitamin C (mg)	23
Vitamin E (mg)	6
Zinc (mg)	0.4

❖ HEALTH & NUTRITION ❖

THERAPEUTIC PROPERTIES

• *Rich in antioxidants*
Orange-fleshed sweet potatoes rival carrots and seaweed for carotenes. Eating high levels of foods rich in carotenes and vitamins C and E is strongly linked with a lower risk of heart disease, stroke, some cancers, and cataracts.

• *Exceptionally high in vitamin E*
Orange-fleshed sweet potatoes contain more vitamin E than any other low-fat food. Vitamin E is linked to many health benefits, including heart and skin health, and male fertility.

• *Excellent potassium source*
A potassium level above that found in most Western-style diets can help prevent and regulate high blood pressure.

• *Good source of iron*
A generous serving of sweet potato is a useful source of iron, especially for vegetarians. Up to one quarter of young women in Western countries are short of iron, causing lower resistance to infection and reduced energy.

Sweet potato
All sweet potatoes are rich in vitamin E, but only the orange-fleshed varieties are rich in carotenes.

HOW MUCH TO EAT

A ½ lb (225g) serving of baked sweet potato supplies an individual's entire daily carotene needs and more than double most people's daily vitamin E requirement. A ½ lb (225g) portion of baked sweet potato also has up to half of the recommended daily potassium intake for an adult, and provides 2g iron, equivalent to 25% of a man's daily requirement and 15% of a woman's. For a protective effect, a helping of foods rich in carotenes, such as sweet potato, is advised at least every other day.

The beta-carotene level of sweet potatoes can be judged by the brightness of their orange color

❖ IN THE KITCHEN ❖

CHOOSING & STORING
Look for sweet potatoes that feel firm and are smooth-skinned. Sweet potatoes do not need to be peeled before they are used because their skin is very thin: scrubbing them thoroughly is enough. Store sweet potatoes in a cool, dark, airy place or in the refrigerator's vegetable drawer.

COOKING & EATING
Sweet potatoes have a distinctive, sweet, chestnutlike flavor. Score them once or twice and bake them in their skins for about one hour at 375°F/190°C. Sweet potatoes are delicious as a side dish with main courses, or on their own with a dollop of cream cheese or sour cream.

RECIPES

Warm Walnut Dip with Grilled Vegetables 105
Sweet Potato Chips 126

BILBERRY

THE FRUITS of the *Vaccinium* family include bilberries, which are known as wild blueberries, and blueberries. These berries deserve to be eaten more often. Today it is easier to do so because farmed berries are more widely available. Blueberries and bilberries have a unique refreshing flavor.

KEY NUTRITIONAL VALUES

per ¼ lb (100g) raw blueberries

Calories (kcal)	30
B vitamins	Good range
Fiber (g)	1.8
Vitamin C (mg)	17

❖ HEALTH & NUTRITION ❖

THERAPEUTIC PROPERTIES

• *Bilberry flavonoids strengthen the blood capillaries and improve circulation* This property may help prevent and treat problems such as chilblains, broken veins, varicose veins, and poor circulation in diabetics.

• *Bilberry extract has been shown to help a range of eye problems* Studies have shown that bilberry extract taken in combination with 20mg of beta-carotene a day may improve adaptation to light and night vision.

• *May help the body resist illness* Bilberry anthocyanin flavonoids have antioxidant, anti-infective, and anti-inflammatory actions. Blueberry anthocyanins have not yet been tested.

• *Counters urinary tract infections* Blueberries contain the same compound that in cranberries prevents the main bacteria that cause urinary tract infections from gaining a hold on the bladder wall.

• *Traditionally used to treat diarrhea* Eating blueberries or bilberries, fresh or dried (stewed or as a tea), is an old remedy for diarrhea.

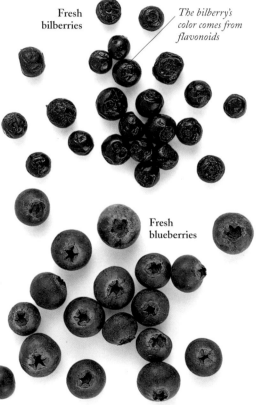

Fresh bilberries

The bilberry's color comes from flavonoids

Fresh blueberries

HOW MUCH TO EAT

Any amount of bilberries, whether eaten raw or cooked, will help strengthen the capillaries or small blood vessels. To prevent or treat ailments, naturopaths suggest a daily serving of the relevant fruit or 2 small glasses of juice or a few glasses of tea made from ½ oz (15g) dried or 2oz (60g) fresh berries to 1 cup (250ml) boiling water.

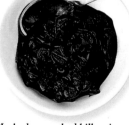

Mashed, uncooked bilberries *make a delicious relish or spread, which can also be eaten on its own, or used in sweet and savory dishes. Freeze until ready to use.*

❖ IN THE KITCHEN ❖

 CHOOSING & STORING Fresh bilberries and blueberries are at their best in late summer and store well if they are chilled. They can easily be made into juice in a food processor. Frozen, bottled, canned, and dried berries are a useful standby for other times of the year. Fresh berries taste better when they are eaten at room temperature.

COOKING & EATING Plain bilberries and blueberries are delicious on their own or mixed with other fruits in a salad. They are traditionally added to pancakes and muffins. Bilberries and blueberries are soft fruit and should only be cooked for a few minutes to retain their fresh flavor. The cooked fruit appears to retain its therapeutic benefits.

RECIPES

Red Fruit Soup 99
Summer Pudding 129
Kissel 133
Oat Bran Muffins (variation) 137

CRANBERRY

HEALTH BENEFITS

*Prevents and treats
urinary tract infections*

◆

*Supports resistance
to disease*

◆

*Small amounts may benefit
kidney stone sufferers*

CRANBERRIES HAVE BEEN valued as a food and medicine for centuries. Native Americans used them for blood poisoning. Cranberries belong to the same family as bilberries. They keep well and were once an important source of vitamin C in winter. One of their best features is their gorgeous red color.

KEY NUTRITIONAL VALUES

per ¼ lb (100g) raw cranberries

Calories (kcal)	15
Fiber (g)	3
Iron (mg)	0.7
Vitamin C (mg)	13

❖ HEALTH & NUTRITION ❖

THERAPEUTIC PROPERTIES

• *Helps prevent and treat urinary tract infections, particularly cystitis in women*
The most common bacteria causing urinary tract infections, *Escherichia coli*, thrives by attaching itself to the walls of the intestines and bladder. An unidentified substance in cranberry discourages the adhesion. In tests, drinking commercial cranberry juice regularly reduced the amount of *E. coli* in urine. For example, of 60 people with urinary tract infections who drank 2 cups (450ml) of juice daily for 21 days, 44 improved. A smaller amount of berries or juice, such as half a cup daily, can help guard against infection starting, even in regular sufferers.

• *Can help the body's defenses*
Cranberries are antiviral and anti-fungal (but not against *Candida albicans*, which causes yeast infections).

• *May aid kidney stone sufferers*
For those with kidney stones, small amounts of cranberries may help lower levels of calcium in urine, so less is present for stone formation.

Fresh cranberries *are best sweetened by mixing them with other sweeter fruits, instead of sugar.*

HOW MUCH TO EAT
To guard against urinary infections, eat about 3oz (75g) fresh cranberries a day or drink 1¼ cups (300ml) of juice (at least 33% pure juice). If treating a urinary infection, eat 6oz (170g) cranberries a day or drink 1½–2 cups (340–500ml) of juice. For urinary infections, eating the fruit is preferable. Most juice drinks are high in added sugar.

Cranberry juice

··········· *Important note* ···········
Cranberries are high in oxalates, which, in the long term, can encourage kidney stones. Do not eat large amounts regularly.

❖ IN THE KITCHEN ❖

CHOOSING & STORING
Homemade cranberry dishes are best. Commercial varieties are usually high in added sugar. Buy cranberries fresh, frozen, or dried. The properties of cranberries are heat-stable, but are less active in the juice and dried fruit. Fresh cranberries keep for weeks if chilled and also freeze well. Use straight from the freezer, unthawed.

COOKING & EATING
One of the most traditional ways of eating cranberries is in a tangy sauce, which complements meat, game, and oily-fish dishes. Cranberry sauce can either be sweet, like a preserve, or made with less sugar as a salsa. Chopped or puréed cranberries add zip and color to sweeter fruits, such as pears, peaches, melon, or kiwi.

RECIPES
Red Fruit Soup 99
Cranberry & Apricot Compote 132
Cranberry Fruitcake 136
Cranberry Orange Relish 141

ORANGE

ONE OF THE MOST RELIABLE food sources of vitamin C, oranges are usually eaten raw, so no nutrients are lost in cooking. Vitamin C is not the only virtue of oranges: fiber, fruit flavonoids, and oil all add to their value. Although orange juice is seen as a healthy shortcut, eating the whole fruit is better.

HEALTH BENEFITS

Supports the body's defenses

♦

May cut risk of some cancers

♦

Can help lower blood cholesterol

♦

Aids capillary circulation

KEY NUTRITIONAL VALUES

per ¼ lb (100g) oranges weighed with seeds and peel

Calories (kcal)	26
Calcium (mg)	33
Fiber (mg)	1.2
Folic acid (mcg)	22
Potassium (mg)	110
Vitamin C (mg)	38

❖ HEALTH & NUTRITION ❖

THERAPEUTIC PROPERTIES

• *Oranges combine vitamin C and flavonoids to help the body's defenses*
Vitamin C is vital for resistance to infection, both as an antioxidant and in its role in improving iron absorption. Oranges combine vitamin C with flavonoids, such as hesperidin, which seem to strengthen the vitamin's antioxidant powers.

• *Anticancer potential*
In many studies, people who eat more oranges and other citrus fruits have lower rates of some cancers, especially of the stomach. The fruit may block the possible transformation of nitrates and nitrites in foods, especially smoked foods, into nitrosamines associated with stomach cancer.

• *Pectin helps lower cholesterol*
Oranges provide pectin, a form of soluble fiber that helps reduce blood cholesterol, especially "bad" LDL-type cholesterol.

• *Can improve small blood vessel strength*
Flavonoids and vitamin C in oranges help maintain cell wall strength, aiding capillary circulation.

Pectin is found mainly in the skin around each segment and in the peel

Whole fruit *has more health benefits than orange juice.*

HOW MUCH TO EAT
Any amount of orange helps resistance to illness. One study showed a substantial drop in the risk of cancer for those eating ¼ lb (100g) of citrus fruit a day. The peel and oil are as valuable as the fruit flesh. Freshly squeezed orange juice is high in vitamin C, potassium, and folic acid but cannot replace the benefit of eating the whole fruit.

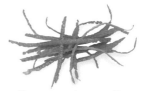

Orange zest *is an excellent way to eat more of the fruit peel, which is richest in beneficial orange oil. Use slender strands of zest to garnish salads and savory dishes and to decorate desserts.*

❖ IN THE KITCHEN ❖

CHOOSING & STORING
Ripe, juicy fruit feels heavy for its size. Fruit that is less ripe contains more pectin. Blood oranges have more carotenes. If using the zest or peel, choose organic or unwaxed fruit, or scrub with warm soapy water and rinse well to help remove pesticide residues. Peeled or stored oranges quickly lose their vitamin C content.

COOKING & EATING
Orange dishes – for example, sliced oranges in liqueur – are convenient and need little added sugar. Marmalade and citrus relishes are good ways of eating the fruit peel. Fresh orange zest adds flavor, color, and tang to salads and many cooked dishes. Eating fresh oranges with smoked foods is a healthy habit.

RECIPES
Munkazina Salad 109
Cranberry Orange
Relish 141

PINEAPPLE

A DELICIOUS FOOD, and one we should enjoy more often, pineapple contains powerful bromelain enzymes. More than 800 research studies have been carried out on the action of these enzymes and show that they can help healing, reduce inflammation from many causes, and improve digestion.

HEALTH BENEFITS

Can help reduce inflammation and speed tissue healing

◆

Helps digestion

◆

Discourages dangerous blood clots

◆

May help angina

KEY NUTRITIONAL VALUES

per ¼ lb (100g) raw pineapple

Calories (kcal)	41
Potassium (mg)	160
Vitamin C (mg)	12

❖ HEALTH & NUTRITION ❖

THERAPEUTIC PROPERTIES

• *Lessens time and degree of inflammation*
The anti-inflammatory action of pineapple is not understood; one theory is that bromelain enzymes block the prostaglandins that play a part in swelling. These enzymes have been used with dramatic success to treat rheumatoid arthritis and to speed tissue repair as a result of injuries, diabetic ulcers, and general surgery. Bromelain enzymes are present in raw pineapple or freshly squeezed juice, although they are more diluted than the enzymes used in research.

• *Enzymes break down protein*
Pineapple enzymes act specifically to break down protein, helping to ease digestion.

• *Reduces blood clotting and may also help remove plaque from arterial walls*
A tendency to form blood clots, which can block an oxygen-carrying blood vessel, is a key factor in heart attacks and strokes. Pineapple enzymes limit this tendency and studies suggest that they may improve circulation in those with narrowed arteries, such as angina sufferers.

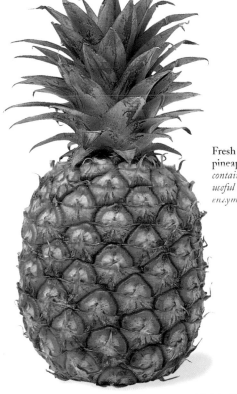

Fresh pineapple *contains useful enzymes.*

HOW MUCH TO EAT
It is impossible to know how much enzyme activity a pineapple has because the action varies according to the different types and may also be affected by growing conditions and ripeness. Eating fresh pineapple often, however, certainly has beneficial effects.

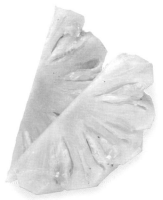

Pineapple slices
The core of the fruit can be eaten as well as the softer flesh.

❖ IN THE KITCHEN ❖

CHOOSING & STORING
Pineapple enzymes are killed by cooking the fruit and pasteurizing the juice. Fresh fruit and freshly squeezed juice retain their health bonus. Pineapples stop ripening once they are picked, so choose fruit that already smells sweet. Large pineapples are a much better value than small ones because the ratio of flesh to skin is much higher.

COOKING & EATING

Peeling a fresh pineapple is as easy as preparing a melon. There is no need to core the fruit. Pineapple complements many foods, from meat and fish to cheese and other fruit. As a marinade, pineapple tenderizes meat and in turn helps the body digest it. However, pineapple quickly curdles cream, custard, and yogurt.

RECIPES
Pineapple Fondue 130
Pineapple Salsa 138

HEALTH BENEFITS

*Discourages blood clots and
stimulates circulation*

♦

*Clears airways congested
due to coughs and colds*

♦

Aid to digestion

♦

May relieve pain

♦

Raises calorie-burning rate

CHILI PEPPER

CHILI CUISINE DOES NOT DESERVE its
reputation for burning your mouth. Whatever
your preference, chilies come in a wide
range of flavors and degrees of heat. They
need not dominate food and can be used
subtly, to deepen flavor. Frequent chili
eaters often grow to like their food hotter.

KEY NUTRITIONAL VALUES

*per ⅓ oz (9g) typical fresh red
chili, weighed whole*

Calories (kcal)	3
Beta-carotene (mcg)	410
Vitamin C (mg)	22.5

*Chilies only make a negligible
contribution to energy, vitamin,
and mineral requirements because
of the small quantities eaten.*

❖ HEALTH & NUTRITION ❖

THERAPEUTIC PROPERTIES

• *Reduces tendency to form blood clots*
Strokes and some heart attacks are
precipitated by the formation of a
blood clot, which can block an oxygen-
carrying blood vessel. Eating hot chilies
regularly stimulates circulation and
may help prevent blood clots.

• *Helps flush out the body's airways*
Eating hot chilies causes sweating
and makes the eyes water and the
nose run. The warming, stimulant
action of chilies increases mucus
flow and helps clear congestion in the
airways, which eases coughs and colds.

• *Stimulates digestion*
Chilies can increase gastric acid,
which helps ensure that there is
enough acid to kill most bacteria in
food, and enable efficient digestion.

• *Relieves pain for some people*
Chilies can have a numbing effect
on pain, which is not yet understood.

• *Temporarily raises calorie-burning rate*
Eating less than 1 teaspoon (3g) of
chili sauce with a meal raised the rate
of calories used in volunteers by an
average 25% for some hours.

*Capsaicin, the source
of chili's heat, is
highest in the seeds*

Fresh
green chili

Fresh red
chili

Crushed dried chilies

Hungarian paprika

HOW MUCH TO EAT
Hotter chili peppers contain
more capsaicin, the source
of their warming, stimulant
properties, so less needs
to be eaten for medicinal
benefits. For example, about
2 teaspoons of fresh jalapeños
a day is enough to benefit
the circulation or the body's
airways. If eaten regularly,
any amount will contribute
to preventive health benefits.

·········· *Important notes* ··········
*Heavy use of chilies may increase
the risk of stomach cancer. Do not
touch the eyes or any cuts when
handling fresh chilies. Opinion
varies on whether people with
peptic ulcers can tolerate chilies.*

❖ IN THE KITCHEN ❖

CHOOSING & STORING
The spiciness and heat of chilies
vary widely. Hungarian paprika and Spanish
pimento are the mildest and are pretreated
to reduce their capsaicin content. Dried
chilies and chili powder retain their
pungency, some beta-carotene, and little
or no vitamin C, lessening their antioxidant
activity. Chili sauces are a good standby.

COOKING & EATING
Hot regions have a wide-ranging
repertoire of chili cuisine, so there are many
recipes to choose from. Chilies are usually
seeded before being added to a recipe. If
a dish tastes too hot, it can be "cooled" by
adding a substantial amount of plain yogurt.
Before adding chilies to a recipe, assess
their "heat" by a quick taste.

RECIPES
Hot & Sour Soup 99
Spiced Chicken Coconut
Soup 101
Salsas 138–9
Zhoug Relish 139

GARLIC

GARLIC IS PROBABLY the best-known healing food, its benefits praised by both the ancient Greeks and Egyptians and now supported by modern research. Its health advantages are wide-ranging because it aids the circulation and resistance to infection, which in turn affect many aspects of the body's health.

HEALTH BENEFITS

Fights infection

Helps heart health

May lower risk of stroke

Aids good circulation

Can help diabetics

May reduce risk of cancer

KEY NUTRITIONAL VALUES

per ⅓ oz (9g), about 2 large cloves

Calories (kcal)   9

Garlic only makes a negligible contribution to energy, vitamin, and mineral requirements because of the small quantities eaten.

❖ HEALTH & NUTRITION ❖

THERAPEUTIC PROPERTIES

• *Antibiotic action against infectious agents*
Garlic can subdue a range of bacterial, viral, and fungal infections, such as flu, colds, cold sores, gastroenteritis, and yeast infections.

• *Reduces raised blood cholesterol*
Many studies confirm this effect. Eating 1–2 fresh garlic cloves a day can decrease blood cholesterol levels by about 10%.

• *Helps blood flow freely*
Studies show that garlic helps dilate blood vessels and reduces the risk of blood clots, which can block blood vessels, leading to a heart attack or stroke.

• *Lowers high blood pressure*
Several studies confirm that valuable drops can be produced by moderate amounts of garlic.

• *Lowers blood sugar levels*
Reducing the rise in blood sugar in response to food helps some diabetics.

• *Anticancer action*
Chinese population studies have shown that those who usually ate the most garlic had less than half the risk of stomach cancer of those who ate the least garlic.

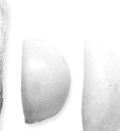

Garlic cloves
Raw garlic is probably the most active form therapeutically.

Purple-skinned garlic bulb

HOW MUCH TO EAT
The effect of 1–2 fresh garlic cloves, or ⅓ oz (9g), a day on heart health is substantial after several weeks. Studies using much more garlic have not had greater results. Similar amounts are suggested to help prevent and fight infections. Since the health benefits of garlic are linked to the smell of its volatile oil, high-heat cooking that disperses this oil will reduce the benefits.

Crushed garlic cloves
Crushing garlic releases its oil, allowing beneficial sulfur compounds to form. To capture these volatile compounds, eat garlic as soon as possible after crushing or chopping.

❖ IN THE KITCHEN ❖

CHOOSING & STORING
Fresh garlic is the only form that can be relied upon to provide therapeutic benefits, as well as the freshest flavor. Processed forms, such as garlic paste and dried or powdered garlic, are not as beneficial as fresh and can easily acquire a rancid flavor. Keep fresh garlic covered, but not airtight, in the refrigerator.

COOKING & EATING
Garlic is an ideal ingredient in dishes that might otherwise seem oily or fatty. It balances the taste just as it balances your body's digestive response. Garlic and olive oil, or garlic and lamb, are examples of delicious combinations. Eating parsley or chewing a coffee bean are traditional antidotes for garlic breath.

RECIPES
Forty-Clove Garlic Chicken 117
Zhoug Relish 139
Garlic Salsa 139
Roast Garlic Salsa 139

GINGER

FRESH GINGER IS a warming, pungent spice and a cornerstone of Asian cuisine. "Stem" is a more exact description than "root" because the part of this tropical plant that we eat is the underground stem. Ginger keeps many of its healing properties when dried, but fresh ginger is superior for use in cooking.

HEALTH BENEFITS

Helps prevent nausea

◆

Relieves indigestion and flatulence

◆

Discourages blood clots

◆

Stimulates circulation and combats colds and coughs

◆

May relieve rheumatism

KEY NUTRITIONAL VALUES

per 1oz (25g) piece fresh ginger

Calories (kcal)   10

Ginger only makes a negligible contribution to energy, vitamin, and mineral requirements because of the small quantities eaten.

❖ HEALTH & NUTRITION ❖

THERAPEUTIC PROPERTIES

• *Combats nausea and motion sickness*
Ginger is as effective as conventional drugs for preventing nausea, but cannot stop existing nausea.

• *Aids digestion and helps relieve flatulence*
Ginger stimulates bile and helps relax colic and quell flatulence.

• *Reduces tendency to blood clots*
In tests, ginger is even more effective than garlic or onion in discouraging the formation of blood clots, which can block blood vessels, causing a stroke or heart attack.

• *Helps fight colds and coughs*
Ginger has a warming, stimulant effect on the circulation, which aids the body in dislodging phlegm and congestion.

• *May help rheumatic pain, stiffness, and swelling*
A 1992 Danish study confirmed the traditional Ayurvedic use of ginger for rheumatism and arthritis. No side effects were reported. Ginger may work by blocking inflammatory substances.

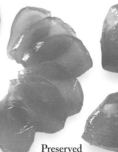

Sliced fresh root

Ground ginger

Fresh ginger

Preserved ginger

HOW MUCH TO EAT

The amount of fresh and dried ginger used in cooking is sufficient for beneficial effects on health. Only ½ teaspoon (1g) of dried ginger, or a small piece of fresh or preserved ginger, is needed for motion sickness. For rheumatism, try eating 1¾ oz (50g) of cooked or 2½ teaspoons (5g) raw fresh ginger a day for at least 3 months. Excess ginger may cause itchiness in and around the bladder opening. If this occurs, eat less.

❖ IN THE KITCHEN ❖

CHOOSING & STORING
Store fresh ginger, wrapped, in the refrigerator to prevent it from drying out or becoming moldy. It should keep for a few weeks and also freezes well. To retain the flavor of dried ginger, buy small amounts and store in an airtight container in a dark, cool place. Preserved ginger in syrup and pickled ginger are useful standbys.

COOKING & EATING
Ginger's scent and "bite" give spicy warmth to curries, stir-fries, many Chinese fish recipes, and a wealth of cold-weather warmers, such as gingerbread and ginger cakes and hot toddies. Ginger goes well with some fruits, most famously melon, but also pears, bananas, and peaches. It is also delicious with ice cream.

RECIPES
Baked Ginger Bananas 129
Gingerbread with Almonds 135

TEA

TEA IS OFTEN criticized for being a stimulant, but it is a mild one, and is proving to have useful health benefits, providing we do not drink too much of it. Green, oolong, and black tea are made from the leaves of the same plant. The process of making teas darker reduces, but does not remove, their health value.

HEALTH BENEFITS

May reduce risk of cancer

May lower risk of heart disease

Counters blood clotting and raised blood pressure

Helps prevent tooth decay

Combats flu virus

KEY NUTRITIONAL VALUES

per 2 tsp (5g) tea

Fluoride (mg)   0.2–0.5

Tea only makes a negligible contribution to energy, vitamin, and mineral requirements.

❖ HEALTH & NUTRITION ❖

THERAPEUTIC PROPERTIES

• *Antioxidant flavonoids*
Antioxidant flavonoids in tea can hinder potential cancer-causing substances such as nitrosamines associated with smoked food and the residues of nitrate fertilizers. A study in Japan showed that an area with a high rate of drinking green tea had lower rates of stomach cancer.

• *May protect heart health*
Drinking tea discourages blood clots, a major cause of heart attacks and stroke. It tends to reduce both cholesterol and fat levels in the blood and can help reduce raised blood pressure. In 2 studies, those who drank the most tea had the fewest heart attacks.

• *Rich food source of fluoride*
In low-fluoride areas, drinking 2–3 cups of tea a day can reduce tooth decay.

• *Antiviral effect*
Tea's traditional use as an antiviral against flu is supported by research.

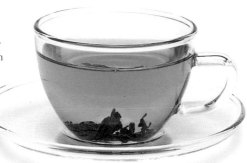

Green tea has a stronger antioxidant action and less caffeine than black tea.

Green tea   Black tea   Oolong tea

HOW MUCH TO DRINK
Tea varies widely in its content of tannins and other flavonoids, with green tea highest, followed by oolong, then black. Adding milk to tea inactivates some of the protective tannins and fluoride. Tea made from 1½–2½ teaspoons (3–5g) of leaves is considered a protective daily amount.

·········· *Important notes* ··········
Drinking too much tea is counter-productive. Excess fluoride mottles the teeth and excess caffeine causes insomnia. Drinking scalding tea has been linked to cancer of the esophagus, and any tea drunk with meals reduces the absorption of iron from food, see p. 25.

❖ IN THE KITCHEN ❖

CHOOSING & STORING
For therapeutic benefits, green tea is the best choice, followed by oolong and green jasmine teas, and then Earl Grey, Indian, and Ceylon black teas. Green and black tea can be mixed. Decaffeinated tea retains its tannins and other flavonoids. Buy tea leaves in small quantities and store in an airtight container in a dark, cool place.

COOKING & DRINKING
In order to minimize the amount of caffeine in tea, throw away the first cup from the leaves, which contains the highest amount. The following cups will contain more of the tannins and other flavonoids. In addition to its use as a hot or cold drink, tea adds a delicious flavor to breads, fruit compotes, sorbets, and sherbets.

RECIPES
Shrimp in Green Tea 116
Earl Grey Tea Bread 136

OATS

OATS ARE ONE OF the most valuable staple foods. Unlike most grains, there is no refined version of oats, so their natural nutritional benefits are retained. Compared to other grains, oats supply more linoleic acid, B vitamins (especially when eaten raw in muesli), vitamin E, protein, and soluble fiber.

HEALTH BENEFITS

Can reduce blood cholesterol

◆

Traditional nerve soother

◆

Help stabilize blood sugar levels

◆

Suitable for gluten-free diets

◆

Ease constipation

KEY NUTRITIONAL VALUES

per 1½ oz (42g) raw rolled oats

Calories (kcal)	160
B vitamins	Good source
Total fat (g)	3–4
• *polyunsaturated (g)*	1.5
• *monounsaturated (g)*	1.3
Fiber (g)	2.8
Folic acid (mcg)	25
Vitamin E (mg)	0.7

❖ HEALTH & NUTRITION ❖

THERAPEUTIC PROPERTIES

• *Can lower blood cholesterol levels*
In a group eating a low-fat diet, those who ate 1¼–1½ oz (35–45g) oatmeal a day had a 3% greater drop in total cholesterol, and a 14% cut in "bad" LDL-type cholesterol after 8 weeks. Other studies had similar results, with most benefit to those with moderately raised levels.

• *Nerve restorative and sedative*
Oats have a traditional reputation for helping the nerves. In a study, withdrawal symptoms in 26 former heavy smokers were eased more by an oat extract than by a placebo.

• *Soluble fiber slows digestion*
Oats slow the absorption of carbohydrate into the bloodstream. This leads to smaller rises and falls in blood sugar, helping some diabetics.

• *Nutritious gluten-free staple food*
A 1995 Finnish study showing that 92 people with celiac disease (who must avoid all gluten) could safely eat oats, suggesting that most celiacs can include oats in their diet.

• *Provide dietary bulk*
Oat fiber eases constipation.

Oat bran can have a dramatic effect on moderately raised cholesterol levels.

Raw oats are treated before rolling to destroy an enzyme that can break down the fat in oatflakes, which can give a bitter, rancid taste.

Cooked oatmeal is a nourishing food that is beneficial to heart health.

HOW MUCH TO EAT
For sedative purposes, eat ½ oz (15g) a day, raw or cooked. To avoid or reduce raised cholesterol levels and steady blood sugar levels, eat 1¾ oz (50g) oatmeal or rolled oats a day. For a more dramatic effect on cholesterol, eat up to 3oz (75g) oat bran a day, only until levels fall, then reduce to 1¾ oz (50g).

·········· *Important note* ··········
Amounts greater than those suggested should not be eaten regularly. Oat bran is high in phytic acid, which limits the absorption of calcium, iron, and zinc from other foods.

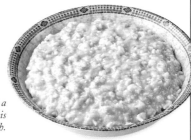

❖ IN THE KITCHEN ❖

CHOOSING & STORING
Partly because of their high polyunsaturated fat content, oats are more vulnerable to rancidity than other grains. Store oats in an airtight container in a cool, dark place and use within a few months. Rolled oats and oat bran are more versatile for cooking than oatmeal, but the latter is more traditional for cooked oatmeal.

COOKING & EATING
Oats are quick and convenient to cook and should be used more often. Rolled oats make tastier cooked oatmeal than instant oat cereal. Rolled oats can be used on their own, or mixed with oat bran, to bind ingredients, for example, in meatballs, or to thicken soups and casseroles. Adding oats to pastry gives extra texture.

RECIPES
Real Muesli 131
Oat Bran Muffins 137

SUNFLOWER

SUNFLOWER SEEDS ARE far richer in vitamin E than any other common food. Once dismissed, vitamin E is now firmly linked with lower risk of heart disease, some cancers, and cataracts. Sunflower seeds are also a prime source of the essential fatty acid linoleic acid, vital to many health functions.

HEALTH BENFITS

Can lower heart disease risk

◆

May help prevent angina

◆

Provides antioxidant defense against cancer and cataracts

◆

Prevents muscle damage after intense exercise

KEY NUTRITIONAL VALUES

per 1oz (28g) sunflower seeds

Calories (kcal)	163
Total fat (g)	13
• *linoleic acid (g)*	8
• *saturated fat (g)*	1
Fiber (g)	6
Vitamin B₁ (mg)	0.4
Vitamin E (mg)	11

❖ HEALTH & NUTRITION ❖

THERAPEUTIC PROPERTIES

• *Rich natural source of vitamin E and linoleic acid, which benefit the heart*
A World Health Organization study suggests that a low level of vitamin E is the most important risk factor in deaths from heart attack. People with low vitamin E levels are nearly 3 times more likely to develop angina. Increasing linoleic acid decreases both total and "bad" LDL-type cholesterol, which helps prevent narrowing of the arteries. Linoleic acid also discourages blood clotting.

• *Anticancer potential*
People who eat more foods rich in the antioxidants beta-carotene and vitamins C and E have lower levels of cancer and are less vulnerable to cataracts as they get older.

• *Prevents damage caused by exercise*
Exhaustive exercise increases the concentration of free radicals in the body, which can lead to muscle damage unless ample vitamin E is present to prevent oxidation.

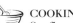

Sunflower seeds

Seeds are dried before eating

HOW MUCH TO EAT
Eating just 1oz (28g) or about 2 tablespoons of sunflower seeds a day will roughly double most people's current vitamin E intake, a major step toward the optimum intake of 40–60mg a day suggested by antioxidant experts.

············ *Important note* ············
Eating seeds or oils that are rancid, either because of overheating or poor storage, increases the risk of the formation of free radicals.

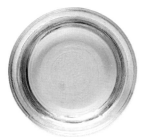

Unrefined sunflower oil *has more flavor than refined oil and loses no nutrients in processing.*

❖ IN THE KITCHEN ❖

CHOOSING & STORING
Be sure sunflower seeds and products are not too old or rancid. Its high vitamin E content makes sunflower the best choice for spreads. Freshly hulled seeds are an even gray color, not yellow or brown. Store seeds and oil in an airtight container in a cool, dark place and use quickly. Toasted seeds retain their vitamin E.

COOKING & EATING
Sunflower seeds add a nutty sweetness to many dishes, from salads to rice dishes and baking. Toasting them enhances this flavor, but limit cooking time to 1–2 minutes in a heavy-bottomed pan over low heat to avoid damaging their essential fatty acid. Break up the seeds a little in a mortar and pestle to release their flavor.

RECIPES
Sunflower Green Salad 112
Sunflower, Apple & Apricot Crumble 133

HEALTH BENEFITS

*Helps lower blood fats
and cholesterol*

◆

*May reduce heart
disease risk*

◆

Anti-inflammatory action

◆

*Good source of nutrients for
those with small appetites*

WALNUT

RICH AND AROMATIC IN flavor, the walnut kernel is a useful nonanimal source of alpha-linolenic acid and linoleic acid, the two essential fatty acids that the body cannot make itself, see p. 19. Increasing the ratio of these polyunsaturated fats to saturated fats in the diet has substantial health benefits.

KEY NUTRITIONAL VALUES

per 1oz (28g) freshly shelled kernels

Calories (kcal)	193
Total fat (g)	19
• *linoleic acid (g)*	9
• *alpha-linolenic acid (g)*	0.9
Iron (mg)	0.81
Selenium (mcg)	5.3
Vitamin E (mg)	1.1
Zinc (mg)	0.75

❖ HEALTH & NUTRITION ❖

THERAPEUTIC PROPERTIES

• *Helps maintain heart health*
Linoleic acid can reduce blood cholesterol levels. Linoleic acid and alpha-linolenic acid, an omega-3 fatty acid, discourage blood clots. Two large-scale diet surveys showed that people who ate walnuts had a lower risk of coronary heart disease. In a third, walnuts lowered blood fats, including cholesterol, and blood pressure levels. Drops in cholesterol can be substantial within 4 weeks, with a rise in HDL "good" and a drop in LDL "bad" types.

• *Omega-3 fatty acids have an anti-inflammatory action*
Omega-3 fatty acids have been used successfully to reduce the severity of rheumatoid arthritis and itchy, scaly skin conditions.

• *Concentrated source of nutrients*
The high calorie concentration in walnuts and their substantial nutrient levels make them good for people with small appetites, such as convalescents.

Unripe, green fruit ("wet" walnuts)

Freshly shelled walnuts *are delicious eaten raw or cooked and are a concentrated source of nutrients.*

HOW MUCH TO EAT
Five walnuts, or 10 halves, (about 1oz/28g) supply total linoleic acid needs for a day, and over half the basic alpha-linolenic requirement. Do not overdo it: eating large amounts of polyunsaturated fats increases your need for vitamin E, see p. 19, and can be fattening. Walnut oil also supplies essential fatty acids, but turns rancid even more easily than walnuts.

---------- ***Important note*** ----------
Never eat walnuts that taste bitter. This means oxidation has started with possible harmful effects.

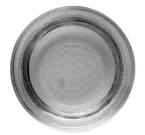

Unrefined walnut oil

❖ IN THE KITCHEN ❖❖

CHOOSING & STORING
Select fresh walnuts in the shell or vacuum-packed walnut kernels, not chopped or ground walnuts, which easily turn rancid when the cut surface reacts with oxygen in the air. Keep walnuts and unrefined walnut oil in an airtight container in a cool, dark place and use quickly. Walnuts in the shell can be frozen.

COOKING & EATING
Freshly shelled walnut kernels, whole or chopped, give a sweet, rich flavor to many recipes, from salads and rice dishes to poultry and fruit desserts. Walnut oil is sweeter than olive oil and wonderful in salads and for use in baking. Avoid strong heating of either walnut kernels or oil as polyunsaturated fats burn and oxidize easily.

RECIPES
Warm Walnut Dip with
Grilled Vegetables 105
Georgian Chicken with
Walnuts 118

YOGURT

ONE OF THE MOST versatile foods, yogurt's long-established reputation as an aid to good health is increasingly reinforced by research. While all yogurt has a high nutritional value, only yogurt which contains "live" bacterial cultures has extra therapeutic benefits. *Lactobacillus acidophilus* is especially valuable.

HEALTH BENEFITS

Helps avoid gastrointestinal and urinary tract infections and yeast infections

♦

Aids recovery from diarrhea

♦

Counters the side effects of antibiotics

♦

Supports the immune system

KEY NUTRITIONAL VALUES

per ½ cup (140ml) serving low-fat plain yogurt

Calories (kcal)	78
Calcium (mg)	210–280
Vitamin B2 (mg)	0.4

❖ HEALTH & NUTRITION ❖

THERAPEUTIC PROPERTIES

• *Protects against some harmful bacteria*
Eating live yogurt made with *Lb. acidophilus* reduces vulnerability to gastroenteritis and yeast infections. Some forms of *Lb. acidophilus* counter common bacteria that cause food poisoning, urinary tract infections, and some peptic ulcers.

• *Speeds recovery from diarrhea*
In clinical trials, children eating yogurt with live *Lb. acidophilus* were twice as likely to recover from diarrhea in 3 days without antibiotics as children given antibiotics. Adults suffering diarrhea and using antibiotics recovered much faster if also given live yogurt.

• *Helps restore gut microflora*
Low levels of healthy microflora in the intestines, which are a side effect of antibiotics, affect the body's ability to fight infection and diarrhea. Eating live yogurt helps restore gut microflora.

• *Stimulates immune defenses*
Yogurt made with live *Lb. acidophilus* stimulates the body cells that fight harmful bacteria and the output of gamma interferon, a substance with antiviral action.

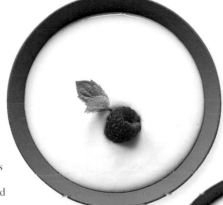

Live yogurt
is not heat-treated. All yogurt is made by growing live bacteria in milk, but if the yogurt is heat-treated, for example, pasteurized, the bacteria are killed.

Whole-milk yogurt
Creamy whole-milk yogurt is higher in fat than most yogurt but is still lower in fat than cream.

HOW MUCH TO EAT
A ½-cup (140-ml) serving of yogurt provides a useful proportion of daily calcium needs and a good range of B vitamins. Many people who cannot digest milk can absorb calcium from yogurt. Yogurt's beneficial cultures cannot survive long in the intestines, so occasional consumption is not as beneficial as eating yogurt every day. For a protective effect against certain harmful bacteria, eat 1 cup (225ml) a day. Yogurt works best if it is eaten the same day as infection begins.

❖ IN THE KITCHEN ❖

CHOOSING & STORING
All types of yogurt are equally rich in calcium. For optimum health benefits, however, choose live low-fat yogurt, either plain, fruit, or flavored varieties. Live kefir, koumiss, and yakult are cultured milk drinks with health benefits equal to those of yogurt with active cultures, but they are less useful for cooking. Store chilled.

COOKING & EATING
The delicate flavor and creamy smoothness of yogurt have traditionally been used to complement many flavors, from spicy cumin seeds to sweet fruit. To obtain the maximum health bonus, it is best to eat yogurt uncooked, since heat kills its helpful cultures. If using yogurt in hot dishes, add it just before serving.

RECIPES

OILY FISH

EATING OILY FISH REGULARLY, whether salmon or a sardine, is one of the best-proven ways to eat for health. Some 800 research papers have linked a wide range of health benefits to the omega-3 fatty acids in oily fish. These include discouraging heart disease and blood clots, and providing anti-inflammatory action. The high vitamin D level of oily fish is valuable to many, and there are plenty of convenient, economical ways to include more oily fish in your diet.

HEALTH BENEFITS

Lower risk of death from heart disease

❖

Can reduce risk of stroke

❖

Help rheumatoid arthritis

❖

May help ulcerative colitis

❖

Can aid inflammatory skin conditions

❖

May reduce risk of cancer

❖

Rich in iodine

KEY NUTRITIONAL VALUES

¼ lb (100g) canned sardines in oil, drained weight

Calories (kcal)	180
Calcium (mg)	21
Iodine (mcg)	37
Iron (mg)	0.4
Omega-3 fatty acids (g)	3.9
Vitamin B$_1$ (mg)	0.23
Vitamin D (mcg)	8.0
Vitamin E (mg)	1.9
Zinc (mg)	0.6

❖ HEALTH & NUTRITION ❖

THERAPEUTIC PROPERTIES

• *Can lower blood pressure, cholesterol, and fat levels, and reduce tendency to blood clots*
In one of several studies, eating canned mackerel 3 times a week for 2 weeks significantly reduced blood pressure and cholesterol levels, which are known risk factors for heart disease and stroke. However, researchers pointed out that those who already ate fish 3 times a week did not benefit more.

• *Reduce risk of death from heart attack*
In a long-term Dutch study, men who ate oily or white fish at least twice a week were less likely to die from heart disease. In a Welsh study of 2,000 men recovering from their first heart attack (who have a higher-than-normal risk of another), half were asked to eat at least 2 portions of oily fish a week. There were 29% fewer deaths in those eating oily fish than the other 1,000 men. The men who ate fish did not have fewer repeat heart attacks, but survived them better. The Dutch study included white fish, so protective effects may not be limited to oily fish alone.

• *Anti-inflammatory action of omega-3 fatty acids can help rheumatoid arthritis*
Eating 4–6 meals with oily fish a week – about 1lb 9oz (700g) in total – is suggested by a research team that found that sufferers of rheumatoid arthritis who were given fish oils had less tender joints and less need for pain relief. Any benefits take several weeks to show.

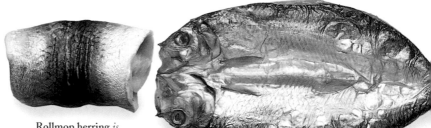

Rollmop herring *is pickled and eaten raw.*

Kipper (smoked herring)

Fresh mackerel

❖ IN THE KITCHEN ❖

CHOOSING & STORING
All varieties of oily fish supply omega-3 fatty acids except canned tuna, which has negligible amounts. Make full use of fresh, smoked, or canned varieties of oily fish: omega-3 fatty acids are reduced by high-heat cooking, but enough survive to be effective. Richest sources of omega-3 fatty acids include mackerel, salmon, kippers, sardines, and herrings. Fish eaten with bones, for example, whitebait or canned sardines, is an excellent source of calcium. Keep both fresh and smoked fish chilled.

COOKING & EATING
The more omega-3 fatty acids you eat, the more vitamin E you need to protect these polyunsaturated fats from oxidation, see p. 19. Use recipes that combine omega-3 fatty acids and extra vitamin E, for example, a smoked mackerel salad dressed with unrefined sunflower oil or a sprinkle of freshly flaked almonds on baked mackerel. When eating smoked fish, add vitamin C to the meal – for example, a good squeeze of lemon – which may help protect against the potentially harmful by-products of smoking.

RECIPES

• *May benefit ulcerative colitis*
Early trials have shown encouraging results. This condition, in which the intestines are inflamed, can be very serious in some people, but it improved in 7 out of 10 sufferers who took fish oil supplements and who had failed to improve with conventional treatment.

• *Good for psoriasis and dermatitis*
Sufferers of psoriasis and dermatitis have reported that fish oils relieve itchiness, scale, and general severity. In a 12-week Norwegian study, the amount of fish oils obtained from a small daily portion of oily fish substantially helped moderate to severe cases of dermatitis. Sufferers who were given an olive oil placebo instead did not improve. Other treatments, such as ultraviolet light for psoriasis, were more effective when combined with eating fish oils.

• *May protect against some cancers*
In animal tests, omega-3 fatty acids raised cancer resistance.

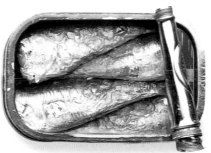

Canned sardines *eaten with the bones are an important source of calcium*

Fresh sardines

Fresh salmon *is a valuable source of vitamin D for people who get little from sunlight on skin, see p. 147.*

HOW MUCH TO EAT
Many experts advise eating at least 2 meals with fish a week, 1 with oily fish. For women, the ideal weekly amount of oily fish is estimated at 4½–13oz (120–380g), and for men it is 5¼–17oz (150–480g). Recent tests have shown that even small amounts of oily fish produce benefits over several months. A US National Heart, Lung, and Blood Institute study suggests that a daily intake of 0.5–1g of omega-3, such as ¼ lb (100g) salmon, could reduce the risk of heart disease in middle-aged men by about 40%. Extra benefits are unlikely if more than 1lb 9oz (700g) a week is eaten.

Whitebait *provide a calcium bonus because they are eaten whole, and are also extremely high in vitamin E.*

············ *Important note* ············
Do not confuse the benefits of oily fish with cod liver oil. Cod liver oil is low in omega-3, but very high in vitamins A and D. Both vitamins can build up in the body, so taking too much cod liver oil can cause an overdose of vitamins A and D.

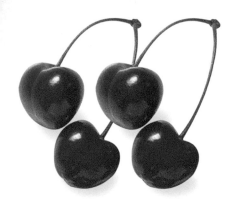
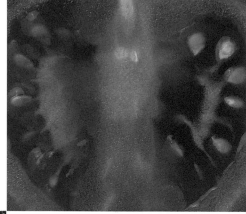
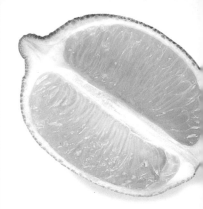
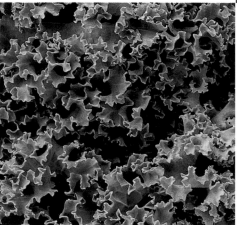
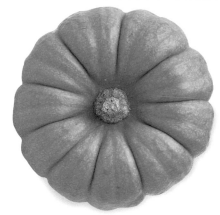
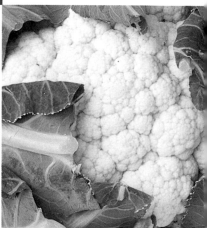
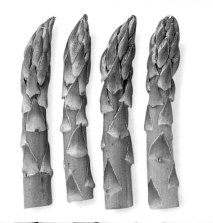
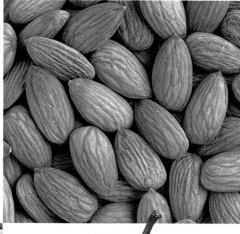
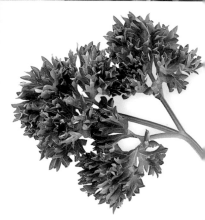
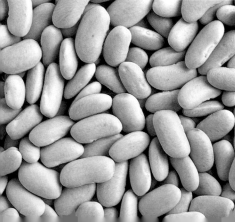
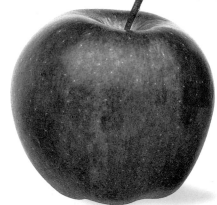
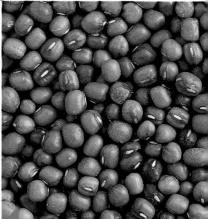

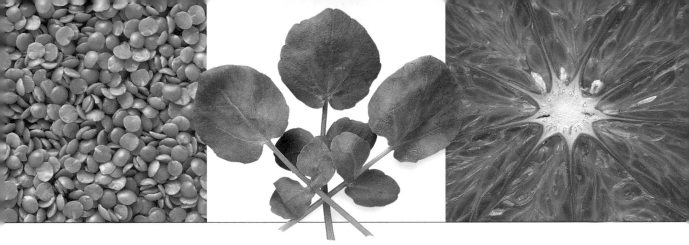

GOOD FOODS

A spotlight on thirty enjoyable foods to

eat more often to protect and support your health.

Their nutritional value and other special

properties can help a wide range of health problems.

Compact profiles equip you with the

practical knowledge to make the most of them.

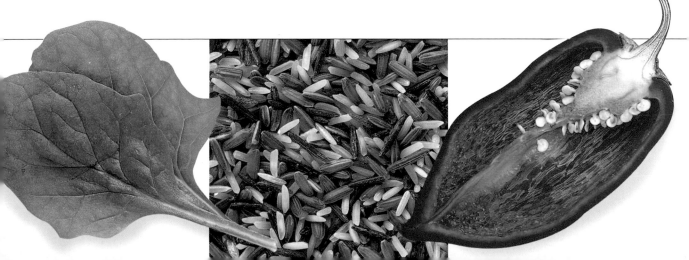

ASPARAGUS

········· HEALTH BENEFITS ·········
- ◆ *Can relieve indigestion*
- ◆ *Diuretic effect*
- ◆ *Traditional sedative*

····· KEY NUTRITIONAL VALUES ·····
per ¼ lb (100g) cooked asparagus

Calories (kcal)	13	Potassium (mg)	110
Carotenes (mcg)	255	Vitamin C (mg)	5
Folic acid (mcg)	74	Vitamin E (mg)	0.56

IT IS GOOD to have reasons to eat this delicious vegetable more often. Asparagus may seem too expensive to eat frequently, but as an ultrasimple, elegant first course, its price compares favorably with many other foods.

❖ HEALTH ❖ & NUTRITION

THERAPEUTIC PROPERTIES
• *Rivals drug treatment of indigestion*
The Ayurvedic herbal use of asparagus for indigestion was tested against a drug commonly used to prevent nausea, hiatus hernia, and heartburn due to gastric acid reflux. Asparagus was similar in effectiveness, without side effects.

Green asparagus *has more vitamins than white.*

• *Traditional diuretic*
Asparagus has long been eaten to stimulate urine production in order to treat fluid retention, and for ailments associated with sluggish digestion, such as rheumatism and arthritis.
• *Reputed to have a sedative action*
Herbalists recommend asparagus to counter colic and heart palpitations.

HOW MUCH TO EAT
Eat freely. Asparagus retains its diuretic effect when cooked. Fresh is best. Frozen and canned asparagus are good alternatives (but canned is high in salt, counteracting its diuretic effect). Green stalks contain a little more carotenes and vitamin C than white.

················ *Important note* ················
Gout sufferers should avoid asparagus. It is high in purines that can raise uric acid levels.

❖ IN THE KITCHEN ❖

CHOOSING & STORING
Two kinds of fresh asparagus are available – green stalks or thicker white stalks. Asparagus toughens during storage; keep it cool, wrapped, and try to use it the same day.

COOKING & EATING
Because asparagus tips cook more quickly than the bases, use a tall, lidded pot (special ones are available) to hold the stalks upright. Cut off any brown or woody stems before cooking.

················ RECIPES ················
Asparagus with Parmesan & Nutmeg 105
Asparagus Frittata 120

CELERY

········· HEALTH BENEFITS ·········
- ◆ *Can help regulate blood pressure*
- ◆ *Diuretic effect*
- ◆ *Traditional soother*

····· KEY NUTRITIONAL VALUES ·····
per ¼ lb (100g) raw celery

Calories (kcal)	7	Sodium (mg)	60
Carotenes (mcg)	50	Vitamin C (mg)	8
Folic acid (mcg)	16	Vitamin E (mg)	0.2
Potassium (mg)	320		

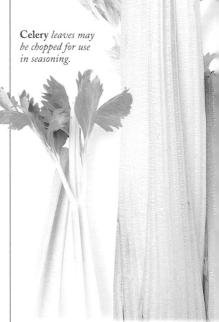

Celery *leaves may be chopped for use in seasoning.*

CELERY WAS GROWN as a medicinal plant long before it was enjoyed as a food. Celery and its relative celeriac (p. 142) are good examples of how you should not underestimate the value of a food just because it is about 90% water.

❖ HEALTH ❖ & NUTRITION

THERAPEUTIC PROPERTIES
• *Helps control blood pressure*
Celery's high potassium content and diuretic effect on the urinary system can help prevent and reduce high blood pressure. In tests, celery lowered blood pressure in animals, and it has been reported to do so in humans.
• *Diuretic effect may help joint conditions*
Celery stimulates urine production, which may be helpful for joint complaints, such as gout, which are related to the body's retention of unwanted substances.
• *Calming effects*
Traditionally, celery has been used to treat nervousness. The essential oil and the seeds contain tranquilizing agents, some of which are also present in the stalks, although the amount has not yet been measured.

HOW MUCH TO EAT

Eat freely. To help lower blood pressure, about 4 stalks a day is the human equivalent of the amount given to test animals. Herbalists recommend cooked as well as raw celery. Greener celery has more vitamin C, folic acid, and carotenes.

❖ IN THE KITCHEN ❖

CHOOSING & STORING
Choose crisp, untrimmed, preferably organically grown celery, because it is prone to high nitrate levels encouraged by nitrate fertilizers. Store celery, wrapped, in the refrigerator.

COOKING & EATING
Celery complements cheese, nuts, and game dishes, such as venison. Keep the outer stalks and leaves for soups or casseroles. Remove strings from the outer stalks with a vegetable peeler.

RECIPES
Waldorf Salad 110
Celery Amandine 120

CRUCIFEROUS VEGETABLES

HEALTH BENEFITS

- *Strong link to a lower risk of cancer*
- *Can help prevent heart disease and stroke*
- *May cut risk of cataracts*
- *High in many nutrients*
- *Counter anemia and risk of spina bifida*
- *Can help regulate blood pressure*

KEY NUTRITIONAL VALUES

per ¼ lb (100g) raw Brussels sprouts

Calories (kcal)	42	Iron (mg)	0.7
Calcium (mg)	26	Potassium (mg)	450
Carotenes (mcg)	215	Vitamin C (mg)	115
Fiber (g)	4	Vitamin E (mg)	1
Folic acid (mcg)	135		

LIKE CABBAGE and broccoli, other cruciferous vegetables such as kale, Brussels sprouts, cauliflower, kohlrabi, mustard greens, collard greens, rutabagas, and turnips are linked with lower rates of cancer. Crucifers, named after the cross-shape of their 4-petaled flowers, are among the best all-around nutrition boosters.

❖ HEALTH & NUTRITION

THERAPEUTIC PROPERTIES
- *Likely to reduce the risk of several cancers*
Large-scale population surveys, plus experimental laboratory testing, suggest that eating plenty of crucifers may halve the risk of several cancers, notably of the lung and colon, but not of the breast, ovary, uterus, or prostate. The link seems to be due to their combination of antioxidants and indole glucosinolates, see p. 23.
- *Rich in antioxidants*
In surveys, people who eat more of foods rich in the antioxidants vitamin C, vitamin E, and carotenes have a lower risk of heart disease, stroke, and cataracts.
- *Rich nutrient source*
Leafy green crucifers are one of the best low-calorie sources of several vitamins and minerals.
- *Top suppliers of folic acid and iron*
Folic acid and iron help prevent and correct anemia. Ample folic acid cuts the risk of spina bifida. The vitamin C level of crucifers helps iron absorption.
- *High in potassium*
Most crucifers are rich in potassium, which can help prevent and regulate high blood pressure.

HOW MUCH TO EAT
Try to eat some raw or lightly cooked cruciferous vegetables 2–3 times a week. A 5¼ oz (150g) serving of green leafy crucifers can supply at least 50% of the most generous recommendation of folic acid for an adult and 25% of the level of folic acid suggested for a woman planning a pregnancy. A 5¼ oz (150g) serving of collard greens can supply 30% of the daily iron requirement for women in their reproductive years.

Important note
Cruciferous vegetables reduce iodine absorption. People who eat more than 3–4 servings a week should ensure they eat iodine-rich foods, especially if they live in an area with low soil iodine.

❖ IN THE KITCHEN ❖

CHOOSING & STORING
Choosing fresh, green leafy crucifers is important. The outer leaves are sweeter, which will encourage you to eat more of their high levels of carotenes and vitamin C. Store, wrapped, in the refrigerator and eat as soon as possible.

COOKING & EATING
In addition to vegetable gratin dishes and oriental stir-fries, explore main dishes combining cruciferous vegetables with nuts and seeds. Carminative spices, such as dill and fennel, help reduce flatulence.

RECIPE
Cauliflower Amandine 120

Green leafy cruciferous vegetables *such as kale are nutritional superfoods.*

Brussels sprouts *are especially rich in folic acid.*

Cauliflower

FENNEL

◆ *Traditional aid to digestion*
◆ *Can ease colic and intestinal cramps*
◆ *May help regulate hormone levels*
◆ *Traditionally used for coughs*
◆ *Can help prevent and counter high blood pressure*

···· KEY NUTRITIONAL VALUES ····

per ¼ lb (100g) raw fennel

Calories (kcal)	12	Vitamin C (mg)	5
Folic acid (mcg)	42	Zinc (mg)	0.5
Potassium (mg)	440		

THE CLEAN, FRESH taste of fennel seems to tell you it must be good for you. Although low in calories, fennel is one of the most satisfying vegetables to use in a main course. The active ingredients of fennel oil are found in the seeds and, to a lesser extent, in the fennel stems that we eat as a vegetable.

❖ HEALTH ❖ & NUTRITION

THERAPEUTIC PROPERTIES

• *Helps digestion*
Fennel is well known for its ability to relieve gas, flatulence, and belching. Fennel oil is included in many gripe medicines for children.

• *Antispasmodic*
Fennel, particularly the seeds, has an antispasmodic effect, easing colic and painful intestinal cramps.

• *Mimics the female hormone estrogen*
Fennel has long been used for its estrogenic effects – for example, to encourage the production of breast milk and to stimulate menstruation. In 1938, the estrogenic action of fennel oil, which is richest in the seeds but is also present in the fronds and stems, was confirmed. This action may ease menopausal symptoms and may help prevent conditions related to estrogen excess, see pp. 86–7.

• *Relieves wheezing*
Syrup made with fennel oil is a long-established expectorant that can help clear coughs.

• *Rich in potassium*
For people eating a typical Western diet, a higher-than-average intake of potassium can help prevent and regulate high blood pressure.

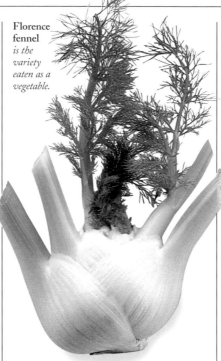

Florence fennel is the variety eaten as a vegetable.

HOW MUCH TO EAT
Eat bulb, stems, and fronds freely. A 7oz (200g) cooked serving supplies 20–30% of an adult's daily potassium requirement. Herbalists recommend a maximum of 1 teaspoon of seeds a day.

················· *Important note* ·················
Do not eat fennel seeds during pregnancy. They may stimulate contractions in the uterus.

❖ IN THE KITCHEN ❖

CHOOSING & STORING
Look for fatter bulbs, which are a better value. Store bulbs, wrapped, in the refrigerator. Keep seeds in an airtight container in a cool, dark place.

COOKING & EATING
Fennel has a delicate aniseed flavor and is delicious raw or cooked. For a main course, allow 1 bulb per person. Use the feathery foliage as a garnish. To release the flavor of the seeds, warm for 1–2 minutes in an ungreased pan over low heat and crush.

··············· RECIPES ···············
Warm Walnut Dip with Grilled Vegetables 105
Fennel à la Grecque 107

PEAS

◆ *May help reduce heart disease risk*
◆ *Help stabilize blood sugar and energy levels*
◆ *Richest food source of vitamin B1*
◆ *Outstanding all-around food*

···· KEY NUTRITIONAL VALUES ····

per ¼ lb (100g) cooked fresh peas

Calories (kcal)	69	Protein (g)	6
Carotenes (mcg)	250	Vitamin B1 (mg)	0.7
Fiber (g)	5.1	Vitamin C (mg)	16
Folic acid (mcg)	27	Zinc (mg)	0.7
Iron (mg)	1.6		

PEAS ARE ONE of the most useful all-around foods, especially as frozen peas retain a high level of nutrients. Just as high in protein as other legumes, peas also have the vitamins of vegetables.

❖ HEALTH ❖ & NUTRITION

THERAPEUTIC PROPERTIES

• *Rich in soluble fiber linked to lower cholesterol levels*
Peas are rich in soluble fiber. Eating more foods that are rich in soluble fiber has been shown to reduce cholesterol levels, especially "bad" LDL type.

• *Slow down digestion, giving a steadier flow of blood sugar and energy levels*
Foods rich in soluble fiber stay in the stomach longer, giving a more gradual rise and fall of blood sugar levels and so helping to keep energy levels steady.

• *High in vitamin B1 (thiamin)*
Peas are the richest food source of vitamin B1, containing even more than liver. Borderline thiamin intake can easily occur in people under stress, the elderly, and heavy drinkers, or in those who are dependent on prepared foods. In a study of 80 healthy Irish women aged 65–92, 70% typically ate 0.8mg of vitamin B1 a day, which should satisfy their needs. Yet those who were given more vitamin B1 had improved sleep, appetite, and cheerfulness, compared to those taking a placebo.

• *Unique range of vitamins and minerals*
Peas rival liver as the food rich in the most nutrients, but are more popular. Like liver, peas are a protein-rich food, high in iron, zinc, folic acid, and other B vitamins, but low in fat, with vitamin C, carotenes, and high fiber.

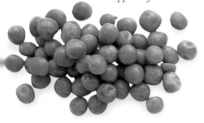

Fresh garden peas

Peas, *whether fresh or frozen, are a top supplier of thiamin.*

PUMPKINS & SQUASH

········ HEALTH BENEFITS ···········
◆ *Antioxidant protection*
◆ *May lower risk of cancer*

····· KEY NUTRITIONAL VALUES ·····
per ¼ lb (100g) baked winter squash

Calories (kcal)	32	Vitamin C (mg)	15
Carotenes (mcg)	3,255	Vitamin E (mg)	1.8
Potassium (mg)	280		

ACORN, BUTTERNUT, and hubbard are just a few of the beautifully shaped varieties of orange- and yellow-fleshed winter squash. Pumpkins are closely related. All are resistant to drought and are symbols of fertility every harvest. The orange and bright yellow flesh of pumpkins and winter squashes is the source of their health benefits.

❖ HEALTH
& NUTRITION ❖

THERAPEUTIC PROPERTIES
● *Strong antioxidant protection*
High levels of the antioxidants vitamins C and E and carotenes in food are strongly linked to a lower risk of cancer, heart disease, stroke, and cataracts.
● *Lower cancer risk*
In several studies of diet and how it relates to cancer, some of the foods eaten more of by those who stay free of cancer are pumpkins and winter squashes. This link occurred in studies as far apart as Australia (in cases of skin cancer), the US (the overall cancer risk for older people), and France (comparing the diet of men with and without bladder cancer).

HOW MUCH TO EAT
For a protective effect, a helping of foods rich in carotenes, such as pumpkins and winter squashes, is recommended at least every other day.

HOW MUCH TO EAT
A 5¼ oz (150g) serving of lightly cooked fresh peas supplies an adult's total daily thiamin needs. Lightly cooked frozen peas supply about 40%. A ¼ lb (100g) serving of lightly cooked fresh or frozen peas supplies about 50% of daily fiber needs, and about 16% of a woman's daily iron requirement and 25% of a man's. Canned peas are not recommended. They lose most of their nutrients and have added salt. Snow peas, sugar snap peas, and petits pois have much less thiamin than garden peas, although they are good sources of iron and fiber.

❖ IN THE KITCHEN ❖

CHOOSING & STORING
Look for fresh peas with crisp, tender pods and store, wrapped, in the refrigerator. Use within 2 days.

COOKING & EATING
Fresh or thawed frozen peas are a delicious and colorful ingredient for salads, or can be added to stir-fries and soups just before serving.

··················· RECIPES ···················
Vegetable Chowder 103
Salmon Kedgeree 116
Broccoli Stir-Fry 121

❖ IN THE KITCHEN ❖

CHOOSING & STORING
Pumpkins and winter squashes are hard-skinned and keep for months. They should be firm and smooth. Canned pumpkin is a good standby.

COOKING & EATING
Pumpkins and winter squashes are equally at home in sweet and savory dishes, from pumpkin pie to curried soup. For easy peeling, cut both into segments and bake beforehand.

··················· RECIPES ···················
Vegetable Chowder 103
Warm Walnut Dip with Grilled Vegetables 105
Spiced Winter Squash 125

This winter squash *has bright yellow flesh, the color provided by its carotenes.*

RED PEPPER

HEALTH BENEFITS

- *Antioxidant protection*
- *Rich source of vitamin C*

KEY NUTRITIONAL VALUES

per ¼ lb (100g) raw red pepper

Calories (kcal)	32	Vitamin C (mg)	140
Carotenes (mcg)	3,840	Vitamin E (mg)	0.8
Niacin (mg)	1.3		

ONE OF THE MOST brightly colored foods, the red pepper is correspondingly high in health value. Peppers become sweeter as they ripen, changing color from green to red.

❖ HEALTH ❖ & NUTRITION

THERAPEUTIC PROPERTIES

- *High in the antioxidants vitamins C and E and carotenes*

Red peppers contain one of the highest concentrations of key antioxidants found in everyday food. People who eat more foods rich in these antioxidants have lower levels of many forms of cancer, as well as of heart disease, stroke, and cataracts.

- *Exceptionally high in vitamin C*

¼ lb (100g) raw red pepper provides more than twice the recommended daily intake of vitamin C, and more than half the 200mg that antioxidant experts suggest may be optimum.

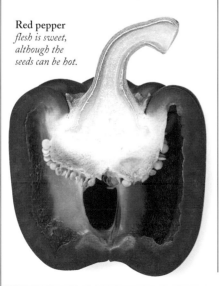

Red pepper
flesh is sweet, although the seeds can be hot.

HOW MUCH TO EAT

Eat freely, either raw or lightly cooked. All peppers are high in vitamin C, but only the red ones are rich in carotenes, especially beta-carotene.

❖ IN THE KITCHEN ❖

CHOOSING & STORING

Look for unwrinkled, shiny peppers. Keep chilled.

COOKING & EATING

The glorious color and sheen of red peppers can transform many bland-looking dishes. Cut peppers as close to serving time as possible, because they lose their crunchiness quickly.

RECIPES

Warm Walnut Dip with Grilled Vegetables 105
Red Pepper Salsa 139

SEAWEED

HEALTH BENEFITS

- *Provides iodine for thyroid health*
- *A useful source of vitamin B12*
- *May help benign breast disease*
- *May have some anticancer action*

KEY NUTRITIONAL VALUES

per 1oz (25g) wakame seaweed, dry weight

Calories (kcal)	18	Magnesium (mg)	118
Calcium (mg)	165	Protein (g)	4
Fiber (g)	12	Vitamin B12 (mcg)	0.6
Iodine (mcg)	4,208	Zinc (mg)	0.4
Iron (mg)	2.9		

SEAWEED IS A traditional food that is being rediscovered not just for its health benefits, but for its subtle flavors. There are many types, such as arame, nori, kombu, hijiki, and wakame, that are essential ingredients of Japanese cookery. Edible Atlantic seaweed includes dulse and purple laver.

❖ HEALTH ❖ & NUTRITION

THERAPEUTIC PROPERTIES

- *Supplies iodine for thyroid health*

Large areas of the world have low soil iodine. Unless inhabitants eat seaweed

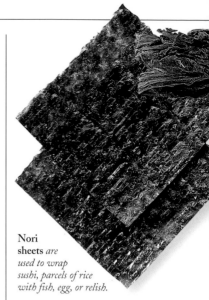

Nori sheets *are used to wrap sushi, parcels of rice with fish, egg, or relish.*

or sea fish, the only reliable food sources of iodine, they are at risk of an underactive thyroid gland. This causes the body's metabolism to slow, leading to tiredness, weight gain, forgetfulness, goiter, and less brain development in the fetus and in infancy. Seaweed contains more iodine than sea fish.

- *Rich plant source of vitamin B12*

Seaweed is virtually the only plant source of vitamin B12, although it is not certain how absorbable the vitamin is from this food.

- *Iodine in seaweed may help benign breast disease*

A Pennsylvania doctor, who noticed that low-iodine areas in the US have high rates of breast cancer, prescribed iodine for 588 women with painful, lumpy breasts (indicating a higher long-term risk of breast cancer). Over a year, 9 out of 10 women had good to excellent results, and 43% felt complete relief from their symptoms.

- *Anticancer action*

In animal tests, seaweed can reduce and delay tumor development, especially of mammary cancers.

HOW MUCH TO EAT

High in sodium, seaweed is best eaten as a flavoring, not in large amounts. Small amounts, such as up to 1oz (25g) dry weight per week, top off iodine levels amply.

Important note

Large amounts of iodine eaten long term – for example, more than 1,000mcg a day – may interfere with thyroid function.

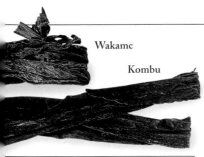

Wakame

Kombu

❖ IN THE KITCHEN ❖

CHOOSING & STORING
Fresh seaweed should be eaten quickly, since it spoils easily. Seaweed is available canned and as laver bread. Dried seaweed, sold in paper-thin sheets or strips, keeps indefinitely if stored in an airtight container.

COOKING & EATING
Nori sheets are eaten dry (slightly heated to crispen if not from a newly opened package) and chopped, to garnish and flavor savory dishes. To reconstitute leafy types of seaweed, soak in water for a few minutes, until softened, then cook or eat in salads in small amounts.

------- RECIPES -------
Suimono Soup 101
Arame, Broccoli & Walnut Salad 110
Shira Ae Salad 111

SPINACH

------- HEALTH BENEFITS -------
- *May reduce risk of cancer*
- *Antioxidant protection*
- *May protect against eye degeneration*
- *Lessens chance of spina bifida*
- *Helps prevent and relieve anemia*
- *Provides plenty of potassium*

----- KEY NUTRITIONAL VALUES -----
per ¼ lb (100g) raw spinach

Calories (kcal)	25	Iron (mg)	2.1
Calcium (mg)	170	Potassium (mg)	500
Carotenes (mcg)	3,535	Vitamin C (mg)	26
Fiber (g)	2.1	Vitamin E (mg)	1.7
Folic acid (mcg)	150		

SPINACH'S FAME as an iron-rich food was due to a misplaced decimal point, multiplying its iron content by ten. Yet the link between spinach and good health is as strong as ever.

❖ HEALTH & NUTRITION ❖

THERAPEUTIC PROPERTIES
- *May lower risk of cancer*
Studies on stomach, skin, lung, prostate, and bladder tumors suggest that people who eat more leafy green vegetables, such as spinach, are likely to have a lower risk of cancer. In a study of 1,271 people aged 66 or over, those who ate the most vegetables rich in carotenes had two-thirds fewer deaths from cancer in the following 5 years, compared with those who ate the least.
- *Rich in antioxidants*
Spinach is high in the antioxidants vitamins C and E and carotenes, which, if obtained from food, are linked in many studies to a lower risk of heart disease, stroke, cataracts, and cancer.
- *May cut risk of age-related macular degeneration (AMD)*
AMD is the main cause of irreversible blindness among adults in Western countries. In a 1994 study in 5 US opthamology centers, people who often ate spinach or collard greens had the lowest risk of AMD, less than those eating plenty of foods rich in carotenes, but not green leafy vegetables.
- *Rich in folic acid*
Spinach, especially raw, is a top source of folic acid, which can lower the risk of having a baby with spina bifida.
- *Useful source of iron*
Spinach is often dismissed as an iron source because it also contains oxalates, which reduce mineral absorption. It is thought this is a short-term effect; in 1 study, the mineral levels of men who ate ¼ lb (100g) spinach every other day sank at first, but were back to normal after 6 weeks.
- *Very rich in potassium*
Ample potassium helps prevent and regulate high blood pressure.

HOW MUCH TO EAT
Spinach should not be eaten every day because it is high in oxalates. However, up to twice a week, preferably raw, is beneficial. Frozen spinach retains more nutrients than fresh spinach that is wilting. Canned spinach retains a substantial amount of nutrients except for folic acid.

-------- *Important note* --------
People with, or who have had, gout or kidney or bladder stones, should avoid spinach due to its high content of oxalates.

❖ IN THE KITCHEN ❖

CHOOSING & STORING
Look for bright green, unwilted spinach leaves. For salads, choose young, small spinach leaves. Chill spinach, wrapped, until ready to use.

COOKING & EATING
Rinse spinach in 2–3 changes of water and cook only with the water left on the leaves after washing. Cover tightly, heat over high temperature until sizzling, then cook for 2–3 minutes until just tender. Drain immediately.

RECIPES
Green Shchi Soup 102
Spinach Amandine 120

Spinach *is rich in antioxidants.*

TOMATO

······· HEALTH BENEFIT ·······

◆ *Antioxidant protection*

····· KEY NUTRITIONAL VALUES ·····

per ¼ lb (100g) raw tomato

Calories (kcal)	17	Potassium (mg)	250
Carotenes (mcg)	1,715	Vitamin C (mg)	17
Fiber (g)	1	Vitamin E (mg)	1.2
Iron (mg)	0.5		

CENTRAL TO the Mediterranean diet, now recognized as one of the healthiest in the world, tomatoes are one of the most versatile food ingredients.

❖ HEALTH ❖ & NUTRITION

THERAPEUTIC PROPERTIES

● *Substantial levels of antioxidants*
Tomatoes contain antioxidants, notably significant amounts of vitamin E, rather less vitamin C, and a small amount of beta-carotene. People who eat more of foods rich in these antioxidants have been shown to have lower levels of several forms of cancer, as well as of heart disease, stroke, and cataracts.

Plum tomato

Garden tomato

Cherry tomatoes

Beefsteak tomatoes

Lycopene, the main carotene in tomato, is the source of its red color

● *May contain other protective substances*
Tomatoes are a good source of the flavonoid substance quercetin, plus a large amount of a carotene called lycopene. Both are being investigated for their potential protective effects.

HOW MUCH TO EAT
Eat freely. Canned tomatoes have nutritional values similar to fresh, except for lower carotenes (200mcg) and vitamin C (12mg). Tomato paste and dried tomatoes are also rich in carotenes and vitamin E. Tomato juice is often high in added salt, which cancels out the value of the potassium.

❖ IN THE KITCHEN ❖

CHOOSING & STORING
All forms of tomatoes are valuable. Canned or dried tomatoes, tomato paste, and juice are all good standbys. Choose products low in salt and, when possible, packed in glass containers. The acidic tomato can leach out the lining from metal or plastic containers.

COOKING & EATING
It is hard to imagine cooking without tomatoes for pasta sauces, pizza, or relishes. Homemade tomato sauce is a delicious low-fat, low-salt alternative to cream sauce. Reduce recipe cooking times when using fresh tomatoes for a better taste (and more vitamins).

··············· RECIPES ···············
Tomato & Wheat Germ Salad 112
Greek Fish Stew 115
Baked Tomatoes 127
Tomato Salsa 139

Watercress contains substantial amounts of B vitamins.

WATERCRESS

··········· HEALTH BENEFITS ···········

◆ *Antioxidant protection*
◆ *May reduce cancer risk*
◆ *Helps prevent and treat infections*
◆ *Counters anemia*
◆ *Helps guard against spina bifida*
◆ *Traditional treatment for eczema*
◆ *Good source of calcium*

····· KEY NUTRITIONAL VALUES ·····

per ¼ lb (100g) raw watercress

Calories (kcal)	22	Potassium (mg)	230
Calcium (mg)	170	Vitamin C (mg)	62
Carotenes (mcg)	2,520	Vitamin E (mg)	1.5
Folic acid (mcg)	200	Zinc (mg)	0.7
Iron (mg)	2.2		

A LONG-ESTABLISHED tonic food for good health, watercress stands out even among other cruciferous vegetables as a food that can offer us a great deal. Watercress has a particular liveliness of flavor – use the leaves in abundance, not just as a garnish.

❖ HEALTH ❖ & NUTRITION

THERAPEUTIC PROPERTIES

● *Concentrated antioxidant protection*
The high levels of carotenes and vitamins C and E in watercress are particularly valuable because it is often eaten raw. A high intake of foods rich in antioxidants has been linked by many studies to a lower risk of cancer, heart disease, stroke, and cataracts. Studies comparing diet records and cancer rates have shown that people who often eat leafy greens, especially crucifers, have lower rates of cancer.

• *Traditional anti-infective*
As well as providing ample folic acid, vitamin C, and zinc, which are required for the efficient functioning of the immune system, watercress has some antibiotic action.

• *Rich in folic acid and iron*
Adequate folic acid is needed for many functions. Watercress is rich in folic acid and iron, which help prevent and correct anemia. Plenty of folic acid reduces the risk of having a baby with spina bifida.

• *Traditionally used for skin problems*
As a "purifying" herb, watercress has long been considered helpful to clear the skin. This may be linked to its mustard oil, which stimulates the circulation and improves the production of gastric acid, which sterilizes bacteria in food.

• *Good source of calcium*
Calcium can be absorbed almost as well from watercress as from milk.

HOW MUCH TO EAT

Eat freely, especially raw. More than 20% of a generous daily intake of calcium for an adult is supplied by ¼ lb (100g). One quarter of the daily recommended amount of folic acid for women planning a pregnancy is supplied by 1¾ oz (50g) of watercress.

···· Important note ····
Do not eat wild watercress. It may harbor watersnails, known to carry the liver-attacking fluke parasite.

❖ IN THE KITCHEN ❖

CHOOSING & STORING
It is almost impossible to prevent fresh watercress from wilting within a few days of picking. Store watercress, chilled, in a bowl covered with a plate. For salads, use within 48 hours.

COOKING & EATING
Watercress must be washed well, in at least 2 changes of water. The leaves and smallest stems are best for salad, but coarser stems can be included if chopped fine. Mix with mild iceberg lettuce or chopped fruit.

···· RECIPES ····
Watercress Soup 103
Munkazina Watercress Salad 109

Unpeeled apples have the most vitamin C and fiber

APPLE

···· HEALTH BENEFITS ····
◆ *Can lower blood cholesterol levels*
◆ *Helps constipation and diarrhea*
◆ *Traditional aid for joint problems*
◆ *Supports general resistance to illness*

···· KEY NUTRITIONAL VALUES ····
per ¼ lb (100g) raw apple

Calories (kcal)	47	Vitamin C (mg)	10
Fiber (g)	1.8	Vitamin E (mg)	0.6
Potassium (mg)	120		

IN TRADITIONAL MEDICINE, apples have been called "the body's broom." This concept of apples as a cleansing food is now supported by our emerging understanding of fiber, antioxidants, and fruit flavonoids.

❖ HEALTH ❖ & NUTRITION

THERAPEUTIC PROPERTIES
• *Can reduce blood cholesterol levels*
Studies show that eating apples can lower blood cholesterol, especially "bad" LDL-type cholesterol. When 30 French men and women added 2–3 apples to their daily diet for a month, 4 out of 5 had a drop in cholesterol, half by more than 10%. Pectin, a soluble fiber in apples, is thought to play a key part in this, but the effect is stronger from eating whole apples than from extracted pectin powder alone.

• *Counters constipation and diarrhea*
The specific combination of fiber types and fruit acids in apples is probably responsible for their well-known ability to prevent and treat constipation. The

liquid-gelling pectin and the natural antiviral properties in apples explain their traditional use for diarrhea.

• *Traditionally used for arthritis, rheumatism, and gout*
The apple's benefits for digestion and the disposal of unwanted substances from the body support its reputation for helping joint problems. This may be due to a combination of actions: fruit acids that improve digestion, the antioxidant effect of the flavonoid quercetin, and pectin's ability to increase elimination.

• *May improve defenses against illness*
Apple pulp, skin, and juice (even when pasteurized) contain substances that destroyed polio and coxsackie viruses in tests of apple juice. In similar tests, fresh apple juice and pectin had some anticancer action.

HOW MUCH TO EAT
Eat apples freely, although more than 2–3 a day does not provide greater health benefits. Apples are best eaten unpeeled, raw, or lightly cooked to provide maximum fiber and vitamin C. Sour and green apples usually have more vitamin C than sweeter or red ones. Canned, stewed apples, dried apples, and apple juice retain fiber, but are vulnerable to oxidation, see p. 96.

···· Important notes ····
Drinking large quantities of apple juice encourages tooth decay and diarrhea, especially in children. Apple juice that has turned brown may encourage carcinogenic compounds.

❖ IN THE KITCHEN ❖

CHOOSING & STORING
Any apples not grown organically should be scrubbed thoroughly with warm, soapy water and rinsed. Store, wrapped, in the refrigerator.

COOKING & EATING
Cooking with sweet apples reduces the need to add sugar. To prevent peeled apples from turning brown, coat them in a little citrus juice.

···· RECIPES ····
Waldorf Salad 110
Winter Pudding 129
Apple Almond Fool 130
Real Muesli 131

APRICOT

········· HEALTH BENEFITS ·········
- *Rich in the antioxidant beta-carotene*
- *Can help regulate blood pressure*
- *High in soluble fiber*
- *Good source of iron*

····· KEY NUTRITIONAL VALUES ·····

per 1¾ oz (50g) dried apricots

Calories	94	Iron (mg)	2
Carotenes (mcg)	323	Potassium (mg)	940
Fiber (g)	3.9		

WHETHER DRIED OR FRESH, apricots have a glorious color. They sweeten food in a nutritious way and fresh apricots provide a useful amount of beta-carotene. Dried apricots are one of the simplest ways to eat more potassium.

❖ HEALTH ❖ & NUTRITION

THERAPEUTIC PROPERTIES
• *Exceptionally high in beta-carotene*
Dark orange fresh apricots are one of the top fruits for beta-carotene. Foods high in this antioxidant are linked to a lower risk of heart disease, stroke, cataracts, and some forms of cancer.

Fresh apricots
Deeper colored fruit have more beta-carotene.

Dried apricots

Unsulfured dried apricot

• *Dried apricots are rich in potassium*
A higher-than-typical Western intake of potassium helps prevent and regulate high blood pressure.
• *Rich in soluble fiber, which steadies blood sugar levels and helps constipation*
Studies have shown that a high intake of soluble fiber steadies blood sugar and energy levels by slowing digestion. It can also help lower cholesterol levels. Dried apricots in particular help prevent and treat constipation.
• *Helps prevent iron deficiency*
A low intake of iron is a common cause of loss of resistance and stamina.

HOW MUCH TO EAT
Eat fresh or dried apricots freely. A handful of dried apricots, or about 1½ oz (40g), supplies around 20% of the suggested daily intake of potassium for adults; and more than 10% of the most generous iron allowance for women in their reproductive years, and almost 20% for men. Eat dried apricots with foods that are rich in vitamin C to help improve iron absorption.

············ *Important notes* ············
Bright yellow or orange dried apricots are preserved with sulfur dioxide, which can cause adverse reactions in some asthma sufferers. The kernels can be toxic.

❖ IN THE KITCHEN ❖

CHOOSING & STORING
Look for firm, bright orange fruit, which is likely to contain more beta-carotene. Unsulfured dried apricots lose most of their beta-carotene. "Ready-to-eat", semi-dried apricots may contain more preservative than fully dried fruit.

COOKING & EATING
Fresh, ripe apricots need only a few minutes simmering. Dried apricots are best cooked in 2 stages. Bring to the boil for 5 minutes and drain. This removes most preservative. Cover with fresh water, boil, and simmer for a further 20 minutes, or until tender. Carotenes are not destroyed by cooking.

············ RECIPES ············
Apricot Almond Fool 130
Cranberry & Apricot Compote 132
Sunflower, Apple & Apricot Crumble 133

BANANA

········· HEALTH BENEFITS ·········
- *Good source of potassium*
- *Can aid stamina in prolonged exercise*
- *Can help relieve constipation and diarrhea*
- *May help sleep and improve mood*

····· KEY NUTRITIONAL VALUES ·····

per ¼ lb (100g) banana weighed with skin

Calories	62	Vitamin B6 (mg)	0.19
Niacin (mg)	0.5	Vitamin C (mg)	7
Potassium (mg)	270		

THE HEALTH BENEFITS of bananas – the ultimate convenience food – change as they ripen. Bright yellow, firm textured bananas have the virtues of starchy foods and give a gentle, long-lasting energy rise. In riper, creamy fleshed bananas most of the starch has turned to sugar, which gives quick energy in exhaustion.

❖ HEALTH ❖ & NUTRITION

THERAPEUTIC PROPERTIES
• *Good source of potassium, whether ripe or less ripe*
Eating more potassium than the typical Western diet provides can help prevent and regulate high blood pressure.
• *Good food for energetic activity*
The starch in less ripe bananas resists digestion and, along with the fruit's soluble fiber, provides a gentler, longer-lasting energy rise than most sweet foods, which is good for stamina. Very ripe bananas are high in sugars. Eaten after 30 minutes of exercise, when muscle energy is exhausted, ripe bananas can improve stamina.
• *Less ripe bananas counter constipation; ripe, sugary bananas help relieve diarrhea*
The starch in less ripe bananas resists digestion, leading to bulkier feces, easing constipation. Very ripe bananas are traditionally used for diarrhea.
• *Ripe bananas may raise mood and help sleep*
Carbohydrates eaten with little protein are known to have a soothing effect by stimulating serotonin, a substance that raises mood, see p. 93. Ripe bananas eaten on their own supply all the ingredients for this reaction: quickly absorbable carbohydrate, serotonin, its precursor tryptophan and vitamin B6.

Ripe bananas *provide rapid energy in exhaustion.*

HOW MUCH TO EAT
Eat freely, but if you eat them between meals brush the teeth as ripe, sugary bananas encourage tooth decay. Eating 1–2 ripe bananas without any other food can produce substantial rises in mood-raising serotonin and may help sleep. Dried bananas are a more concentrated source of potassium, fiber, and energy than the fresh fruit, but are also higher in sugar.

❖ IN THE KITCHEN ❖

CHOOSING & STORING
Most bananas are at their sweetest when the yellow skin has no trace of green and is dotted with brown spots. To slow ripening, keep bananas in the fridge; the skin will turn brown but the flesh will stay firm and cream-colored for a few days.

COOKING & EATING
Foods and flavorings that bananas partner well include walnuts, coffee, ginger, cinnamon, oranges, ice cream, and liqueurs, especially rum. Bananas brown quickly once peeled unless tossed in citrus juice. In recipes without citrus juice, prepare bananas last and add just before cooking.

RECIPES
Baked Ginger Bananas 129
Banana Walnut Tea Bread 137

BLACK CURRANT

········ HEALTH BENEFITS ········
- *Rich in protective antioxidants*
- *Counters urinary tract infections and food poisoning*
- *Helps relieve inflammation*
- *Traditional diuretic*
- *Good source of potassium*

······ KEY NUTRITIONAL VALUES ······
per ¼ lb (100g) raw black currants

Calories (kcal)	28	Potassium (mg)	370
Carotenes (mcg)	100	Vitamin C (mg)	200
Fiber (g)	3.6	Vitamin E (mg)	1
Iron (mg)	1.3		

BLACK CURRANTS HAVE always been recognized as a food with a health bonus. Although their best-known property is a high level of vitamin C, their health benefits are also reflected in their color, like the orange in carrots or the green in cabbage. The dark purple color of black currants comes from flavonoids, see p. 22. These may help strengthen the walls of small blood vessels, leading to many health benefits.

❖ HEALTH & NUTRITION ❖

THERAPEUTIC PROPERTIES
• *Antioxidant protection*
Black currants are very high in vitamin C and also provide significant amounts of vitamin E and carotenes. People who eat more of foods rich in these antioxidants have been shown to have a lower rate of heart disease, stroke, cataracts, and cancer.
• *Rich in anthocyanins*
Anthocyanin flavonoids counter the common bacteria that cause food poisoning and urinary tract infections. The high pectin level of black currants can also help relieve diarrhea, for which the fruit is traditionally used.
• *Anti-inflammatory action*
Anthocyanin flavonoids are anti-inflammatory, which explains why a black currant drink helps relieve a swollen, sore throat and may also be linked to its traditional use for rheumatism. Black currant seeds contain 25–30% gamma-linolenic acid (GLA), a fatty acid. Extracted from the seeds, GLA is used to treat inflammation associated with rheumatism and skin conditions, such as eczema and psoriasis. In theory, the amount of black currants most people eat provides too little GLA to benefit these ailments but traditional use for rheumatism suggests they are worth trying. Grind the seeds to help make the GLA available to the body.
• *Diuretic with a high potassium level*
Diuretics often help those who suffer from high blood pressure and rheumatism, but deplete their potassium levels. Black currants combine a diuretic effect with a high level of potassium.

HOW MUCH TO EAT
Eat freely, either raw, cooked, or in spreads sweetened only with fruit juice. Black currant juice drinks often contain little fruit: check labels.

❖ IN THE KITCHEN ❖

CHOOSING & STORING
Fresh black currants have a short summer season, but freeze well. Keep fresh berries chilled. Look for black currant juice free from additives and sugar.

COOKING & EATING
Enjoy the tart flavor and the color of black currants in fruit desserts, puddings, and fruit salads. The berries need cooking for a few minutes only, until they burst. Some recipes advise straining the seeds and skins from the berries, but they are beneficial to eat.

············ RECIPES ············
Red Fruit Soup 99
Summer Pudding 129
Kissel 133

Black currants
The sharp flavor of black currants adds a refreshing tang to desserts.

CHERRY

◆ *Helps some gout sufferers*

····· KEY NUTRITIONAL VALUES ·····
*per ¼ lb (100g) raw cherries,
weighed with pits*

Calories (kcal)	39	Vitamin C (mg)	9
Potassium (mg)	170		

CHERRIES DO NOT have many claims to fame but they have helped many gout sufferers. Red, purple, and black cherries get their color from anthocyanins, see p. 22.

Cherries *A tea made from the stems is used as a traditional diuretic.*

❖ HEALTH ❖ & NUTRITION

THERAPEUTIC PROPERTIES
• *Can help gout by lowering uric acid levels*
Gout sufferers build up excess uric acid, a natural waste-product of digestion, which forms into crystals in the joints leading to pain and swelling. Eating 15–25 red or black cherries a day has been reported to lower uric acid levels.

HOW MUCH TO EAT
Eat freely. Fresh cherries have a short season, but frozen, bottled, cooked, and canned cherries should have similar effects on uric acid. There is no evidence regarding dried cherries.

❖ IN THE KITCHEN ❖

CHOOSING & STORING Cherries freeze well without blanching or removing the pits.

COOKING & EATING Cherries are best enjoyed raw. They cook in 3–5 minutes, making it easy to remove the pits.

········· RECIPES ·········
Red Fruit Soup 99
Nut & Cherry Pilaf 123

CITRUS FRUITS

········· HEALTH BENEFITS ·········
◆ *Help maintain the body's defenses*
◆ *Likely to reduce risk of some cancers*
◆ *Can lower blood cholesterol levels*
◆ *Assist capillary circulation*
◆ *Useful source of potassium and folic acid*

····· KEY NUTRITIONAL VALUES ·····
*average values per ¼ lb (100g) clementines,
weighed with seeds and peel*

Calories (kcal)	26	Potassium (mg)	92
Calcium (mg)	22	Vitamin C (mg)	19
Folic acid (mcg)	23		

IT IS HARD TO IMAGINE good cooking without lemons and limes, or good eating without the pleasure of grapefruit, tangerines, and clementines. Even if we did not know they are rich in vitamin C, they would draw us with their colors, aroma, and freshness.

❖ HEALTH ❖ & NUTRITION

THERAPEUTIC PROPERTIES
• *Reliable source of vitamin C for the body's defenses*
Vitamin C is needed daily to sustain the body's resistance to infection and its ability to heal wounds. It also has antioxidant and other functions. Flavonoids, found mainly in the peel and the skin around each segment, support the action of vitamin C.
• *Linked to a lower risk of cancer*
In many studies of diet and cancer, people who eat more

Flavonoids and pectin are found in the skin around each segment

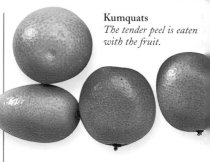

Kumquats
The tender peel is eaten with the fruit.

citrus fruits have lower rates of some cancers, especially of the stomach. Vitamin C is known to block the formation of potentially carcinogenic nitrosamines in the stomach after eating nitrite or nitrates, for example in smoked food. Other elements in citrus fruits are also thought to be protective, including pectin fiber, flavonoids, and citrus oil, which have antioxidant properties. The oil, which is richest in the peel, has shown an antitumor effect in animal tests.
• *Pectin helps reduce blood cholesterol*
Citrus pectin, which is found mainly in the skin surrounding each segment, is a form of soluble fiber and helps reduce blood cholesterol, especially "bad" LDL-type cholesterol.
• *Can improve capillary circulation*
Citrus flavonoids can strengthen capillary walls leading to some anti-inflammatory action.
• *Good source of potassium*
A generous serving of citrus fruits can help balance the Western diet's excess of sodium and so help regulate blood pressure. It can also offset potassium loss caused by taking drugs to control blood pressure.

Lemon and lime *juice, like all citrus juice, prevent the discoloration of peeled fruits and vegetables.*

Clementine

HOW MUCH TO EAT

Eat freely. Even a small quantity of citrus contributes to better body defenses. A generous daily serving of citrus, 2 clementines and ½ grapefruit, for example, provides 15–20% of an adult's daily recommended potassium requirement. Whole peeled fruit, including the membranes between segments, and citrus peel are more valuable than citrus juice.

❖ IN THE KITCHEN ❖

CHOOSING & STORING
Fruit that is less ripe is higher in pectin. For peel or zest, choose organic or unwaxed fruit, or scrub with warm soapy water and rinse to help remove pesticide residues. The redder varieties of citrus fruits, such as pink grapefruit, contain useful amounts of carotenes.

COOKING & EATING
Citrus fruits, whether sweet or sharp, enhance many dishes. Citrus zest adds flavor, color, and freshness to salads and fish dishes.

------------ RECIPES ------------
Honey & Lemon
Cheesecake 131
Lime Salsa 139
Low-Fat Hummus 140

HONEY

------ HEALTH BENEFITS ------
➤ *Can relieve gastric infection*
➤ *May counter ulcer bacterium*
➤ *Helps prevent gastric irritation*
➤ *May help hay fever and related asthma*

----- KEY NUTRITIONAL VALUES -----
per 1oz (25g) honey

| Calories (kcal) | 72 | *Vitamin and mineral content is negligible.* |

HONEY'S HEALING properties have proved more enduring than criticisms that it is just another form of sugar. Most honey is heated to help filter it, delay solidification, and speed jar-filling. To enjoy honey's health benefits to the fullest, use cold-pressed honey and honeycomb, which also have more flavor.

❖ HEALTH ❖ & NUTRITION

THERAPEUTIC PROPERTIES
• *Antibiotic action in the digestive tract*
Cold-pressed honey can destroy a wide range of bacteria in the stomach and intestines, making it a gentle treatment for gastroenteritis and related diarrhea. The antibacterial activity of different varieties of honey varies. For example, studies have shown that cold-pressed New Zealand manuka honey kills 9 bacteria species, including *Helicobacter pylori*, the bacterium now thought to cause many cases of gastric pain and peptic and duodenal ulcers. Tests with heated honey have not had clear results.
• *Protects the stomach lining from irritants*
People who regularly use drugs that irritate the stomach lining, such as aspirin, could benefit from taking cold-pressed honey at the same time.
• *Unfiltered honey may prevent some hay fever (allergic rhinitis)*
There is some evidence that eating the pollen in unfiltered, cold-pressed honey and honeycomb may have a desensitizing effect on hay fever and related asthma. Sufferers are advised to begin eating unfiltered, cold-pressed honey, or honeycomb, daily, in late winter.

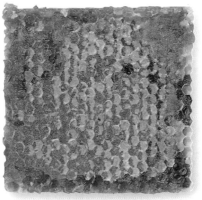

Honeycomb
Beeswax packages honey perfectly, sealing in flavor and usually some pollen.

Manuka honey

HOW MUCH TO EAT
An astonishingly small amount of honey may be enough for therapeutic benefits. For instance, try ½ teaspoon of cold-pressed honey on an empty stomach to help ease peptic ulcers, gastroenteritis, or stomach irritation. A traditional amount for hay fever sufferers is 1 teaspoon of cold-pressed, unfiltered honey, or honeycomb, eaten 3 times a day.

------------ *Important notes* ------------
It is not advisable to give honey to infants under 1 year of age. Adverse reactions, though rare, are not unknown. Honey causes tooth decay as easily as sugar and contains almost as many calories.

❖ IN THE KITCHEN ❖

CHOOSING & STORING
Honey will have been heat-treated unless the label on a jar of honey states that it is cold-pressed, unfiltered, or "raw." The least treated honey is honeycomb. Honey remains liquid or soft longer at room temperature. It keeps indefinitely and there is no need to chill it.

COOKING & EATING
In cold food, honey tastes sweeter than the same weight of sugar and has a superior flavor, so you may not need as much. Since heat reduces the antibiotic properties of honey, add it to dishes after cooking, and, if baking with honey, keep the temperature low.

------------ RECIPES ------------
Honey & Lemon Cheesecake 131
Honey & Mustard Dressing 140

Cold-pressed honey

PARSLEY

········· HEALTH BENEFITS ·········

- *Traditional diuretic*
- *May help kidney function and gout*
- *Antioxidant protection*
- *Counters anemia*
- *Useful source of calcium*

····· KEY NUTRITIONAL VALUES ·····

per ¼ lb (100g) fresh parsley

Calories (kcal)	34	Iron (mg)	7.7
Calcium (mg)	200	Potassium (mg)	760
Carotenes (mcg)	4,040	Vitamin C (mg)	190
Folic acid (mcg)	170		

RECOGNIZED SINCE Roman times as a food with a health bonus, parsley is much too good to use only as a garnish. It improves many dishes and is one of the most nutritionally rich foods, especially since it is usually eaten raw.

❖ HEALTH ❖
& NUTRITION

THERAPEUTIC PROPERTIES

- *Helps the body shed excess fluid*
The diuretic effect of parsley is apparent after eating only 1oz (25g) of fresh parsley. This effect has been traditionally used to treat gout, fluid retention, and poor kidney function.
- *Exceptionally high in the antioxidants vitamin C and carotenes*
People who eat more of foods rich in these antioxidants are likely to have a lower risk of cancer, heart disease, stroke, and cataracts. In 2 studies, parsley leaves restricted the effects

of some known cancer-provoking substances.

- *Combines anti-anemia nutrients*
Just 1oz (25g) parsley provides more iron than a ½ lb (200g) pork chop. The high iron content is combined with a high level of folic acid, also needed for making red blood cells, and vitamin C, which improves iron absorption.
- *Good source of calcium*
Parsley is a useful nondairy source of calcium, especially for anyone who eats few dairy products.

HOW MUCH TO EAT
Eating about 1oz (25g) of fresh parsley a day is one of the simplest ways to improve your intake of iron, calcium, and folic acid, and supplies an adult's daily requirement of vitamin C. About 1½ oz (40g) of parsley supplies about 10% of an adult's daily calcium needs.

············· *Important note* ·············
Although parsley is a rich source of folic acid, herbalists advise against eating more than ½ oz (15g) a day during pregnancy, because it is said to stimulate uterine contractions.

❖ IN THE KITCHEN ❖

CHOOSING & STORING
There are 2 main types of parsley, curly-leaf and flat-leaf. Both are rich in minerals and vitamins, but flat-leaf tastes stronger. Always wash parsley thoroughly to help remove pesticide residues. Store, wrapped and chilled.

COOKING & EATING
Use fresh parsley lavishly in sauces, soups, salads, and salad dressings. Avoid dried parsley. Chop and add parsley just before serving, to retain its full flavor and nutritional value.

············· RECIPES ·············

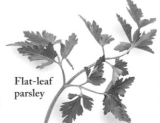

Flat-leaf parsley

Curly parsley

RICE

········· HEALTH BENEFITS ·········

- *Can help prevent chronic Western diseases*
- *Good for bowel health*
- *Encourages stable blood sugar levels*
- *Important source of vitamin B1*
- *Gluten-free and hypoallergenic*

····· KEY NUTRITIONAL VALUES ·····

per 7oz (200g) cooked brown rice

Calories (kcal)	282	Potassium (mg)	19
Fiber (g)	1.6	Vitamin B1 (mg)	0
Iron (mg)	1	Vitamin B2 (mg)	0.0
Magnesium (mg)	220	Zinc (mg)	1
Niacin (mg)	2.6		

RICE IS A STAPLE FOOD for half the world. It is a particularly valuable starchy food to eat more of, especially brown rice. With many varieties and recipes available, rice always offers something fresh and delicious to eat.

❖ HEALTH ❖
& NUTRITION

THERAPEUTIC PROPERTIES

- *Key starchy food*
Experts agree that eating more than the typical Western intake of starchy foods, especially in unrefined forms, helps prevent chronic diseases such as heart disease, high blood pressure, diabetes, and certain cancers, see p. 14
- *May reduce risk of bowel disorders*
Brown rice has less fiber than wheat, but still helps prevent constipation and related disorders. Rice made into gruel with salt is a traditional remedy for diarrhea. In animal trials, rice bran had some effect in preventing bowel cancer. Starch as well as fiber reduces the risk of colon cancer.
- *Steadies blood sugar levels*
Eating rice produces a gentler rise in blood sugar than potatoes or bread. Stable blood sugar helps provide steadier levels of energy, assists diabetic control, and may help prevent excessive weight gain, p. 15.
- *Supplies vitamin B1 (thiamin)*
Borderline thiamin deficiency, see p. 145, is common in people eating a Western diet. Eating brown rice helps boost thiamin levels.
- *Gluten-free and unlikely to cause allergy*
Rice is a safe staple food for anyone who reacts badly to eating wheat.

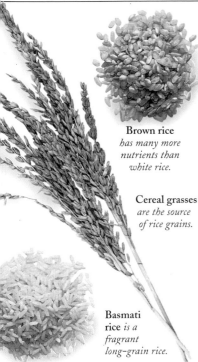

Brown rice *has many more nutrients than white rice.*

Cereal grasses *are the source of rice grains.*

Basmati rice *is a fragrant long-grain rice.*

HOW MUCH TO EAT

International consensus is that complex carbohydrate foods, such as rice, should provide about half the daily calorie intake and be eaten regularly, see pp. 12–13. Refining and milling processes strip away the nutrient-rich outer layers of rice, so try to eat brown rice in preference to white. A 7oz (200g) serving of cooked brown rice supplies about a third of an adult's daily thiamin requirement, compared to white rice, which supplies almost none.

❖ IN THE KITCHEN ❖

CHOOSING & STORING
Parboiled or converted white rice retains slightly more nutrients than ordinary white rice. Brown basmati rice is the quickest-cooking brown rice. Store rice in an airtight container in a cool, dark place.

COOKING & EATING
Once cooked, rice keeps for up to 2 days if covered and chilled. Cooked rice does not freeze well.

RECIPES
Salmon Kedgeree 116
Nut & Cherry Pilaf 123

WHEAT

HEALTH BENEFITS
- ✦ *Can help prevent heart disease*
- ✦ *Protects intestinal and bowel health*
- ✦ *May reduce risk of breast cancer*
- ✦ *Can ease menopausal symptoms*
- ✦ *Important source of selenium*

KEY NUTRITIONAL VALUES
per ¼ lb (100g) whole-wheat bread

Calories (kcal)	215	Potassium (mg)	230
Fiber (g)	5.8	Vitamin B$_1$ (mg)	0.3
Iron (mg)	2.7	Vitamin B$_2$ (mg)	0.1
Niacin (mg)	4.1	Zinc (mg)	1.8
Pantothenate (mg)	0.6		

THE SEED of life for most people in the world, wheat is also the biggest crop. There are many low-fat ways to eat wheat, including in bread and cakes made with whole-wheat flour, as pasta, and grains, such as couscous and bulgur.

❖ HEALTH ❖ & NUTRITION

THERAPEUTIC PROPERTIES
- *High value starchy food*
A substantial amount of data shows that a higher intake of starchy foods is associated with a reduced risk of chronic diseases, see *Rice*, p. 66.
- *Provides insoluble fiber*
Insoluble fiber, more than soluble fiber, helps prevent and treat constipation, which is associated with an increased risk of gallstones, diverticular disease, and bowel cancer.
- *Wheat fiber is linked to lower cancer risk*
In several studies, women who ate more grain fiber had a lower risk of breast cancer. Wheat is a source of phytoestrogen lignans, see p. 23, which in studies reduced high blood levels of estrogen and androgen hormones, a risk factor for breast cancer.
- *Can reduce menopausal symptoms*
In Australian studies, eating either 1½ oz (45g) raw unbleached white flour or

Bulgur wheat
grains have more nutrients than white flour and need very little cooking.

crushed wheat grains daily, reduced hot flashes by 25–50% in menopausal women within 12 weeks, and improved other menopausal symptoms.
- *Provides antioxidant selenium*
Wheat grown in selenium-rich soil is a key source of this antioxidant mineral, which is linked to good heart and circulation health.

HOW MUCH TO EAT

Complex carbohydrates such as wheat should ideally provide about half of the daily calorie intake, see pp. 12–13. Eat unrefined wheat in preference to white, refined forms, for example, whole-wheat bread and whole-wheat pasta.

Important notes
Wheat contains gluten, which must be avoided by people with celiac disease. Do not feed wheat to babies under 6 months. Eat wheat bran freely in bread, but avoid it raw or in cereals. It reduces mineral absorption, see p. 25. In excess, it can irritate the bowel.

❖ IN THE KITCHEN ❖

CHOOSING & STORING
Good quality whole-wheat bread needs little or no spread to be delicious. Wheat breakfast cereals lose vitamins and minerals in processing. Store pasta, grains, and flour in airtight containers in a cool, dark place.

COOKING & EATING
Whole-wheat flour can be used to replace white in most recipes. Whole-wheat pasta can be cooked with white; begin it 2–3 minutes earlier.

RECIPES
Summer Herb Salad 111
Tabbouleh 113
Baking Recipes 134–137

Whole-wheat bread

WHEAT GERM

········ HEALTH BENEFITS ········
- *Good for those with small appetites*
- *Antioxidant protection*
- *Supports heart health*
- *Prevents and relieves constipation*
- *Rich in folic acid*

····· KEY NUTRITIONAL VALUES ·····

per 1oz (25g) wheat germ

Calories (kcal)	76	Potassium (mg)	238
Fat (g)	2.3	Protein (g)	6.7
• *omega-3s (g)*	0.1	Vitamin B1 (mg)	0.5
• *omega-6s (g)*	1.3	Vitamin B6 (mg)	0.8
Fiber (mg)	2.4	Vitamin E (mg)	5.5
Folic acid (mcg)	83	Zinc (mg)	4.3
Iron (mg)	2.1		
Niacin (mg)	1.1		

WHEAT GERM IS the most nutrient-rich part of wheat, retrieved after milling white flour. A convenience food, wheat germ needs no preparation, and just a sprinkle of its golden, nutty flakes gives a health boost to any dish.

❖ HEALTH ❖ & NUTRITION

THERAPEUTIC PROPERTIES
- *Concentrated source of nutrients*
Wheat germ is exceptionally rich in vitamins B1, B6, and E, niacin, and folic acid. This small-volume food is especially valuable for people with a small appetite or few calorie needs.
- *Outstanding source of vitamin E*
A higher intake of the antioxidant vitamin E is strongly linked to a lower risk of heart disease, stroke, cataracts, and some cancers.
- *High in fiber*
Wheat germ can relieve constipation, which not only causes discomfort, but can lead to hemorrhoids and bowel disease, such as diverticulitis.
- *Good source of folic acid*
Folic acid helps reduce the risk of having a baby with spina bifida.

HOW MUCH TO EAT
About 1oz (25g) or 2 tablespoons of wheat germ eaten daily supplies about 40% of an adult's vitamin B1 and folic acid needs, and 20% of the daily requirement for women planning a pregnancy. This amount also raises typical vitamin E intake by 50%.

About 1fl oz (25ml) of wheat germ oil supplies almost 40mg vitamin E, close to the 40–60mg daily amount suggested by some experts for high antioxidant protection.

················· ***Important notes*** ·················
Wheat germ is high in phytic acid, which reduces the absorption of its high iron and zinc content. Eating a vitamin C-rich food at the same meal increases iron absorption.

❖ IN THE KITCHEN ❖

CHOOSING & STORING
Use stabilized wheat germ, in which an enzyme that leads to rancidity has been destroyed. Buy it in small amounts and store, chilled, in an airtight container. It is best to store cold-pressed oil in dark glass bottles in the refrigerator. Both the oil and wheat germ should be used within a few weeks and should taste sweet, not bitter.

COOKING & EATING
Sprinkle wheat germ on salads and cooked dishes alike. Use wheat germ oil in salad dressings. If you prefer the flavor of another oil, blend to taste.

················· RECIPE ·················
Tomato & Wheat Germ Salad 112

WHOLE GRAINS

········ HEALTH BENEFITS ········
- *Help prevent heart disease and other chronic diseases*
- *Stabilize blood sugar levels*
- *May help regulate estrogen levels*

····· KEY NUTRITIONAL VALUES ·····

per 2oz (55g) uncooked whole-grain barley

Calories (kcal)	166	Vitamin B1 (mg)	0.16
Fiber (g)	8	Vitamin B6 (mg)	0.3
Iron (mg)	3.3	Zinc (mg)	1.8
Pantothenate (mg)	1.4		

EATING MORE WHOLE GRAIN staples, such as whole barley, kasha, corn, rye, millet, and quinoa is an important step toward achieving a healthy, balanced diet. The variety of whole grains that are now widely available means your culinary repertoire need never be boring.

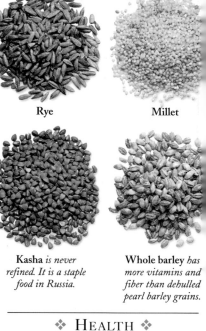

Rye

Millet

Kasha *is never refined. It is a staple food in Russia.*

Whole barley *has more vitamins and fiber than dehulled pearl barley grains.*

❖ HEALTH ❖ & NUTRITION

THERAPEUTIC PROPERTIES
- *Starchy foods aid disease prevention*
A high intake of starchy foods, especially unrefined, is associated with a lower risk of heart disease, high blood pressure, certain cancers, and diabetes, see p. 14.
- *Soluble fiber steadies blood sugar levels*
Whole barley (containing mainly soluble fiber) and whole rye (containing mainly insoluble fiber) have 5–6 times more fiber than most whole grains. These grains produce the gentlest rise in blood sugar after eating, which is especially valuable to diabetics, helping prevent serious side effects and give a steadier flow of energy.
- *Can lower high levels of estrogen*
Eating more high-fiber whole grains can lower high blood levels of the female hormone estrogen, a risk factor for breast cancer, see p. 87.

HOW MUCH TO EAT
Most nutrition experts agree that grains and other starchy foods, preferably unrefined, should provide about half the daily calorie intake, see pp. 12–13. To steady blood sugar and energy levels, choose breads or cereals with whole, chopped, or coarsely milled grains, rather than rolled or fineground.

.... *Important notes* ....
Barley and rye contain some gluten and must be avoided by those with celiac disease. Do not feed barley or rye to babies under 6 months.

❖ IN THE KITCHEN ❖

CHOOSING & STORING
Keep unrefined flours and whole grains chilled, and use quickly.

COOKING & EATING
Most grains are delicious on their own or as an alternative to rice or pasta. Serve them with pasta sauces, fresh herbs, or in salads.

.... RECIPE ....
Oden-Style Stuffed Cabbage 122

BEANS & LENTILS

.... HEALTH BENEFITS ....
- *Can reduce risk of heart disease*
- *Stabilize blood sugar levels*
- *Help prevent or combat anemia*
- *Good source of potassium and folic acid*

...... KEY NUTRITIONAL VALUES ......

per ¼ lb (100g) cooked red kidney beans

Calories (kcal)	103	Iron (mg)	2.5
Calcium (mg)	37	Potassium (mg)	420
Folic acid (mcg)	42	Protein (g)	8.4
Fiber (g)	6.7	Zinc (mg)	1

Pinto beans

Lima beans

DRIED BEANS AND LENTILS, or legumes, have become neglected in the age of convenience foods. But they are well worth eating, especially in place of higher-fat meat or cheese. High in fiber and protein and low in fat, legumes are a key ingredient in many dishes that taste too good to be abandoned.

❖ HEALTH ❖ & NUTRITION

THERAPEUTIC PROPERTIES
• *Lower blood cholesterol levels*
Eating more legumes can substantially reduce blood cholesterol rates, which are a marker for risk of heart disease. In an American study, men with high blood cholesterol levels ate a set diet for 3 weeks, then for the next 3 weeks added 4oz (115g), dry weight, of pinto and navy beans daily, keeping the total calorie and fat intake the same. Blood cholesterol fell by an average 19% and "bad" LDL-type cholesterol by 24%.
• *Rich in soluble fiber*
Many studies confirm that eating legumes, which are rich in soluble fiber, can improve blood sugar control. Legumes slow down the rate of digestion and result in a more gradual rise and fall in blood sugar, steadying energy levels. This is especially valuable for diabetics.
• *Substantial levels of iron and folic acid*
Most legumes can rival white meat or fish for iron, and are also high in folic acid. These help anemia and folic acid reduces the risk of a spina bifida baby.
• *High in potassium*
Eating more potassium than is usual in a typical Western diet can help prevent and regulate high blood pressure.

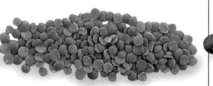

Split red lentils *need no presoaking and cook in 20–25 minutes.*

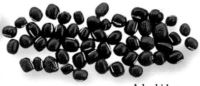

Adzuki beans

HOW MUCH TO EAT
To replace the protein in a meal from meat, fish, eggs, or cheese, use 2oz (55g) beans, dry weight, per person. To reduce cholesterol and blood fat levels, 3½ oz (100g) of legumes, dry weight, a day is ample. A similar effect is found in 16oz (450g) of canned baked beans or fava beans. Canned beans lose most of their vitamins (but not minerals) and have added salt, which counteracts the usefulness of their potassium.

.... *Important notes* ....
Kidney beans must be boiled for at least 10 minutes to neutralize a harmful substance that they contain. Some people of Mediterranean origin suffer from favism, an inherited anemia triggered by eating undercooked fava beans.

❖ IN THE KITCHEN ❖

CHOOSING & STORING
Dried legumes keep well, provided they are stored in an airtight container in cool conditions.

COOKING & EATING
Except for split red lentils, soak legumes overnight before cooking. Cook in fresh water, not the soaking water. Carminative herbs and spices such as dill can help reduce flatulence. Legumes can be added to many conventional dishes, from soups to casseroles, to dilute their fat content.

.... RECIPES ....
Bean Kedgeree 116
Falafel 123
Lima Beans with Sage & Garlic 125
Low Fat Hummus 140

Red kidney beans *mix well into meat dishes, adding fiber and diluting their fat content.*

Black-eyed pea

SOYBEAN

.... HEALTH BENEFITS ....

- *Helps lower risk of heart disease*
- *Eases constipation and improves intestinal health*
- *Steadies blood sugar levels*
- *Rich in iron, calcium, and potassium*
- *Can help ease menopausal symptoms*
- *May reduce risk of breast cancer*

...... KEY NUTRITIONAL VALUES ......

per ¼ lb (100g) cooked soybeans

Calories (kcal)	141	Iron (mg)	3
Calcium (mg)	83	Potassium (mg)	510
Fat (g)	7.3	Protein (g)	14
• *of which 84% unsaturated*		Vitamin E (mg)	1.1
Fiber (mg)	6.1	Zinc (mg)	0.9
Folic acid (mcg)	54		

THE POPULAR perception of soybeans is that they are a worthy but boring food. But soybeans have another side with real appeal – as an ingredient in the delicate dishes of Japanese cuisine and in more robust Chinese dishes.

❖ HEALTH ❖ & NUTRITION

THERAPEUTIC PROPERTIES

- *Helps counter heart disease*
Even people who already eat a low-fat diet can substantially lower their blood cholesterol by replacing some low-fat animal protein with soy products. In tests, people with raised blood cholesterol levels who ate soy products instead of half or all of the animal protein in their diet reduced blood cholesterol by a typical 8–16% over several weeks. Many studies confirm this effect, which is thought to be due to soybeans' particular balance of fiber, fatty acids, and phytoestrogens. Soybeans contain a little alpha-linolenic acid, an omega-3 fatty acid that is linked to better heart health.
- *Rich in soluble and insoluble fiber*
Soybean fiber can prevent and ease constipation, which can lead to diverticulitis and other bowel diseases.
- *Regulates blood sugar levels*
Like other foods high in soluble fiber, soybeans slow down the speed of digestion and the rate of absorption. This produces a gentler rise and fall of blood sugar, which benefits diabetics and helps stabilize energy levels.

- *Good source of iron, calcium, and potassium*
Soybeans provide large amounts of iron, which is absorbed well, unlike iron from most plant foods. Plenty of potassium, above the typical Western intake, can help prevent and regulate high blood pressure. Tofu made with calcium chloride is rich in calcium.
- *Can relieve menopausal symptoms*
Studies show that eating 1½ oz (45g) of soy flour or grits daily can reduce hot flashes and postmenopausal symptoms, such as the loss of bone minerals, within 6–12 weeks. These effects are thought to be due to soy's rich phytoestrogen content, see p. 23. Soybeans are the most estrogenic food known so far.
- *May reduce risk of breast cancer*
Evidence suggests that soybeans have some anticancer activity. One risk factor for breast cancer is a high level of the hormone estrogen in the blood, see p. 87. When women regularly eat foods rich in weak estrogenlike compounds, such as those in soybeans, with fiber, their blood estrogen level falls.

HOW MUCH TO EAT
In order to reduce raised cholesterol levels or to influence hormone levels, eat some tofu, soy flour, or soybeans in place of other protein foods once a day. A 3½ oz (100g) serving of tofu supplies about half of the daily allowance of calcium advised for the highest-needs age group (11–24) for both sexes. Soy milk contains phytoestrogens but little fiber or calcium. Miso, soy sauce, and soybean oil do not have the same benefits as other soy products.

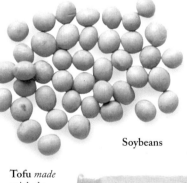

Soybeans

Tofu *made with the setting agent calcium chloride is the richest nondairy calcium source.*

.... *Important notes* ....
Raw soybeans, including soybean sprouts, contain a toxin that must be destroyed by thorough cooking before eating. Because the effects of exposure to estrogenlike compounds in plants early in life are not yet known, the advice pending research is to give soy formula to infants only when there is no other alternative.

❖ IN THE KITCHEN ❖

CHOOSING & STORING
Soybeans keep well in an airtight container. Firm tofu is more useful than soft, unless you are using it for pâté or dressing. Fresh tofu keeps for a few days if chilled. Once unwrapped, immerse it in water.

COOKING & EATING
Soybeans must be soaked for at least 5 hours before cooking, then boiled in fresh water for at least 2 hours until tender. Tofu can be used in similar ways to low-fat soft cheese, in addition to its use in traditional Asian dishes. Use the nutrient-rich liquid as well.

.... RECIPES ....
Suimono Soup 101
Shiro Ae Salad 111
Broccoli & Tofu Stir-Fry 121
Oden-Style Stuffed Cabbage 122

ALMOND

.... HEALTH BENEFITS ....

- *Can lower blood cholesterol levels*
- *May help reduce risk of heart disease*
- *Rich in vitamin E*
- *Useful source of calcium*

...... KEY NUTRITIONAL VALUES ......

per ¼ lb (100g) freshly shelled almonds

Calories (kcal)	612	Potassium (mg)	780
Calcium (mg)	240	Protein (g)	21
Fat (g)	55.8	Vitamin E (mg)	24
• *of which 87% unsaturated*		Zinc (mg)	3.2
Iron (mg)	3		

MANY PEOPLE AVOID nuts, all too aware of their high calorie count. But when you get as much from them as almonds provide, they deserve a place on your shopping list more often.

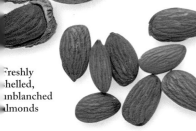

Whole
almonds

Freshly
shelled,
unblanched
almonds

❖ HEALTH ❖ & NUTRITION

THERAPEUTIC PROPERTIES

• *Can help reduce blood cholesterol*
Although almonds are high in fat, it is mainly monounsaturated, p. 19. When volunteers added 3oz (84g) almonds a day to a low-fat diet, they had an average 10% drop in cholesterol, especially "bad" LDL-type cholesterol, within 3 weeks.

• *Rich source of vitamin E*
Almonds are high in vitamin E, which has recently emerged as very protective against death from heart disease when eaten (usually in supplement form) in much higher amounts than the daily adult allowance of 10mg. A leading expert on antioxidants recommends at least 40mg of vitamin E a day. Most people eat under 10mg a day. In 2 large US surveys of diet and heart disease, nut eaters, mainly of almonds and walnuts, had less heart disease.

• *Good source of calcium*
Almonds are one of the richest nonanimal sources of calcium.

HOW MUCH TO EAT

Adding 1oz (25g) of almonds a day to your diet almost doubles the average vitamin E intake. 1¾ oz (50g) almonds a day supplies 10% of the daily calcium requirement for the highest-needs age group (11–24) for both sexes.

❖ IN THE KITCHEN ❖

CHOOSING & STORING
Unblanched almonds have a superior health value compared to blanched almonds in packages. Store in a jar in the fridge, and, once opened, use within a few weeks. Freeze almonds in their shells for out-of-season eating.

COOKING & EATING
Almonds are a versatile food, equally at home in a cake, a salad, or on top of baked fish. Blanching is unnecessary in many recipes. To toast almonds without damaging their oils, heat them gently in an ungreased frying pan for 1–2 minutes.

········ RECIPES ········
Apricot Almond Fool 130
Gingerbread with Almonds 135

LINSEED

········ HEALTH BENEFITS ········
◆ *Key source of omega-3 fatty acids*
◆ *Can ease menopausal symptoms and may help avert breast cancer*
◆ *Prevents and relieves constipation*
◆ *Soothes digestion*

····· KEY NUTRITIONAL VALUES ·····

per ⅓ oz (9g) golden linseed

Calories (kcal)	47	Fiber (mg)	1.6
Fatty acids (g)	2.9	Iron (mg)	0.7
• omega-3s (g)	2.3	Vitamin E (mg)	0.02
• omega-6s (g)	0.7	Zinc (mg)	0.4

A COMMON FOOD in Northern Europe, linseed comes from the beautiful blue-flowering flax plant, from which we also get linen and elements of linoleum. Linseed has extraordinary health benefits and is gaining in popularity because of new, tastier golden linseed.

❖ HEALTH ❖ & NUTRITION

THERAPEUTIC PROPERTIES

• *Rich source of omega-3 fatty acids*
Linseed is one of the few plant sources rich in omega-3 fatty acids, which are known to benefit heart health, the body's defense systems, and inflammatory conditions.

• *Very high in phytoestrogen lignans*
Lignans are among the plant substances that have a weak estrogenlike activity, see p. 23. Tests show that eating 1½ oz (45g) of linseed a day can reduce some menopausal symptoms, such as hot flashes, within several weeks. Lignans may also supplant stronger estrogens, reducing high blood levels

of estrogen, a risk factor for breast cancer, see p. 87. A high intake of fiber also seems to decrease the risk of breast cancer.

• *Gentle, bulk-forming fiber*
In addition to averting constipation, linseed is thought to be prebiotic, encouraging "friendly" intestinal flora, which hinder the development or reabsorption of toxic products of the metabolism.

• *Soothes the linings of the digestive tract*
Linseed contains mucilaginous fiber, which soothes the delicate linings of the stomach and digestive tract. Linseed is a useful form of fiber for people whose digestive systems are easily irritated, such as ulcer sufferers.

HOW MUCH TO EAT

Just 1–2 teaspoons of golden linseed a day is all that is needed for health benefits. To ease digestion or constipation, 2–3 teaspoons a day is helpful. Increase gradually until there is improvement, but do not exceed 1 heaped tablespoon or ⅓ oz (9g) of linseed 2–3 times a day. It is important to drink at least ⅔ cup (150ml) of liquid at the same time.

❖ IN THE KITCHEN ❖

CHOOSING & STORING
Choose organic, golden linseed, which has been lightly cracked, making it easier for the body to extract the nutrients. Store in the refrigerator and use within a few weeks. Linseed oil goes rancid quickly.

COOKING & EATING
Organic golden linseed is delicious sprinkled over cereals, yogurt, and salads, or added to breads and cakes. When using uncooked, add just before eating. Avoid linseed in recipes with long, high-temperature cooking.

·············· RECIPE ··············
Tomato & Wheat Germ Salad 112

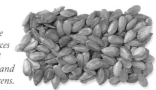

Golden linseed *is one of the richest sources of omega-3 fatty acids and phytoestrogens.*

PUMPKIN SEEDS

⋯⋯⋯ HEALTH BENEFITS ⋯⋯⋯

* *Assist prostate health*
* *Help prevent bladder stones*
* *Useful source of zinc*
* *Support immune system function*

⋯⋯ KEY NUTRITIONAL VALUES ⋯⋯

per 1oz (25g) pumpkin seeds

Calories (kcal)	142	Iron (mg)	2.5
Fat (g)	11.4	Vitamin E (mg)	0.7
• *of which 78% unsaturated*		Zinc (mg)	1.6
Fiber (g)	1.3		

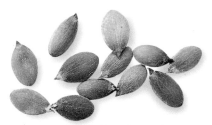

Pumpkin seeds *should be chewed thoroughly to help absorption.*

THE DELICIOUS FLAVOR and semi-crunchy texture of pumpkin seeds adds interest and a fresh green color to cakes or muffins and many savory dishes. Pumpkin seeds give a health bonus of interest to almost everyone.

❖ HEALTH ❖ & NUTRITION

THERAPEUTIC PROPERTIES
• *Tests confirm the traditional use of pumpkin seeds for an enlarged prostate*
In 1990, in a double blind study over 3 months, pumpkin seed extract significantly improved symptoms such as urinary-flow time, quantity, and frequency in sufferers, compared to those given a placebo.
• *Help prevent or relieve bladder stones*
Pumpkin seeds can reduce the formation of calcium oxalate crystals, which can lead to bladder stones. For example, in 1987, in a study of an area in Thailand with a high number of bladder stone sufferers, pumpkin seeds were more effective in reducing crystals than conventional treatment.

• *Richest plant source of zinc*
Zinc is vital to the immune system, for example, to help infection resistance and for wound-healing, growth, and the sense of taste. Marginal deficiency is thought to be common, especially in elderly people and anorexics.

HOW MUCH TO EAT
Just 1¾ oz (50g) of pumpkin seeds a day provides 3.2mg zinc, over a third of the recommended daily intake for a man. Naturopaths recommend that prostate sufferers eat at least 1oz (25g) a day. Zinc is absorbed better from plant foods when eaten with some meat or fish.

❖ IN THE KITCHEN ❖

CHOOSING & STORING
Choose hulled pumpkin seeds that are a uniform green, not brown, which is a sign of rancidity. Store them, chilled, in an airtight container and use within 2 months.

COOKING & EATING
Pumpkin seeds make an enjoyable change from nuts in baking recipes. Sprinkle them over cereal, fruits, salads, and soups. For extra flavor, toast pumpkin seeds in an ungreased frying pan for 1–2 minutes over low heat.

⋯⋯⋯ RECIPES ⋯⋯⋯

Cranberry Fruitcake 136
Oat Bran Muffins (variation) 137

CHICKEN LIVER

⋯⋯⋯ HEALTH BENEFITS ⋯⋯⋯

* *Combats anemia*
* *Speeds recovery from blood loss*
* *Supports immune system function*
* *Provides concentrated nutrition*

⋯⋯ KEY NUTRITIONAL VALUES ⋯⋯

per ¼ lb (100g) sautéed chicken liver, using 6g oil

Calories (kcal)	169	Potassium (mg)	300
B vitamins	Rich source	Retinol vitamin A	
Cholesterol (mg)	350	(mcg)	10,500
Fat (g)	8.9	Vitamin B$_{12}$ (mg)	45
Folic acid (mcg)	1,350	Zinc (mg)	3.8
Iron (mg)	11.3		

THE LESS MEAT you eat, the more valuable chicken liver may be. It is high in iron, folic acid, and zinc – 3 nutrients which many people do not get enough of. Chicken liver is also low in fat, inexpensive, and tastes delicious.

❖ HEALTH ❖ & NUTRITION

THERAPEUTIC PROPERTIES
• *Rich in iron, folic acid, and vitamin B12*
Chicken liver provides an easily absorbed, concentrated source of nutrients needed for making red blood cells to help prevent or treat anemia, or to recover from blood loss, for example, from surgery.
• *High level of zinc*
Chicken liver is rich in zinc, which is essential for growth and the body's immune defenses. Many people who eat little – either to lose weight or due to a lack of appetite, for example, if they are elderly, ill, or anorexic – eat inadequate amounts of zinc.

HOW MUCH TO EAT
Eating chicken liver once a week helps prevent anemia; a little more often is useful to make up for blood loss.

⋯⋯ *Important notes* ⋯⋯
Pregnant women are advised not to eat liver. Excess retinol vitamin A (but not beta-carotene) can cause fetal abnormalities. People who are on low-cholesterol regimens should consult a dietitian before eating chicken liver on a regular basis.

❖ IN THE KITCHEN ❖

CHOOSING & STORING
Fresh chicken liver has a firm texture. Remove any green or yellow pieces. Liver from organic chicken is preferable to ensure that farming chemical residues are not present.

COOKING & EATING
Chicken liver has a delicious melt-in-the-mouth quality (even though it is low in fat), so it can be enjoyed in creamy-tasting pâtés without adding quantities of fat. Chicken stock made with chicken liver has a deep flavor.

⋯⋯⋯ RECIPE ⋯⋯⋯

Chicken Liver & Vermouth Pâté 106

SHELLFISH

········· HEALTH BENEFITS ·········

◆ *Rich in iodine and antioxidant selenium*
◆ *Support immune system function*
◆ *Good for people who eat little*
◆ *Can help heart health*
◆ *May provide anti-inflammatory action*
◆ *Mollusks supply plenty of iron*

····· KEY NUTRITIONAL VALUES ·····

per ¼ lb (100g) cooked mussel meat

Calories (kcal)	104	Selenium (mcg)	43
Calcium (mg)	52	Vitamin E (mg)	1.1
Iodine (mcg)	120	Zinc (mg)	2.3
Iron (mg)	6.8		

THE WIDE VARIETY OF shellfish, from luxurious scallops and lobster to the more affordable mussel or clam, is a never-ending pleasure. Recent research dismisses any link between shellfish and higher blood cholesterol: in fact, it is the contrary, see p. 18. All varieties are strikingly low in calories and fat.

❖ HEALTH ❖
& NUTRITION

THERAPEUTIC PROPERTIES

• *Important source of iodine*
Large areas of the world have low soil iodine. Unless inhabitants eat foods rich in iodine, such as shellfish, they are at risk of disorders of the thyroid gland, which regulates the metabolism.
• *Supply the antioxidant mineral selenium*
Soil levels of this antioxidant, linked to heart and circulation health, vary widely between regions, so shellfish and other seafood are the only reliable sources.
• *Top source of zinc*
Shellfish provide zinc in an easily absorbed form. Even in developed countries, many people would benefit from more zinc, notably those who eat little food – either to lose weight or due to a lack of appetite, for example, if they are elderly, ill, or anorexic.
• *Contain omega-3 fatty acids*
Shellfish are very low in fat, but supply small amounts of omega-3 fatty acids, which are strongly linked with heart health and anti-inflammatory action.
• *May help relieve rheumatoid arthritis*
New Zealand green-lipped mussels may help relieve rheumatoid arthritis. Research on greenshell mussel extract is conflicting, but at least 1 double blind trial has been very positive, with minimal side effects. Sustained popularity suggests many people find it useful. The quantity of mussels that corresponds to a useful amount of extract is not known.
• *Mollusks are very rich in iron*
Clams, oysters, and mussels, are excellent sources of iron, in an easily absorbed form.

HOW MUCH TO EAT

Eat freely. However, eating oysters or other mollusks daily would provide too much zinc and iron. Eating shellfish twice a week helps ensure an adequate supply of iodine, selenium, zinc, and, from mollusks, iron. For instance, ¼ lb (100g) boiled mussel meat supplies 45–68% of the iron, 80% of the iodine, and 15–20% of the zinc of an adult's daily requirements.

Oysters *are by far the richest food source of zinc.*

Mussel

Scallop

Shrimp *are a good source of calcium.*

Crab
A serving provides a useful amount of an adult's daily zinc needs.

·········· *Important note* ··········
People with gout should eat shellfish only rarely. Shellfish are high in purines that can raise uric acid levels.

❖ IN THE KITCHEN ❖

CHOOSING & STORING
Shellfish, especially oysters, clams, and mussels, are the most perishable of foods. Eat or freeze the day purchased. Ready-to-eat or frozen shellfish have often been cooked or glazed in salty water: try to avoid salt elsewhere in the meal.

COOKING & EATING
Shellfish add flavor to salads, soups, or stir-fries. Shellfish are very easy and quick to cook, either steamed, grilled, or baked. Avoid strong, competing flavors that may overwhelm the wonderful, natural flavor of shellfish.

·············· RECIPES ··················
Greek Fish Stew 115
Moules Marinière 115
Shrimp in Green Tea 116

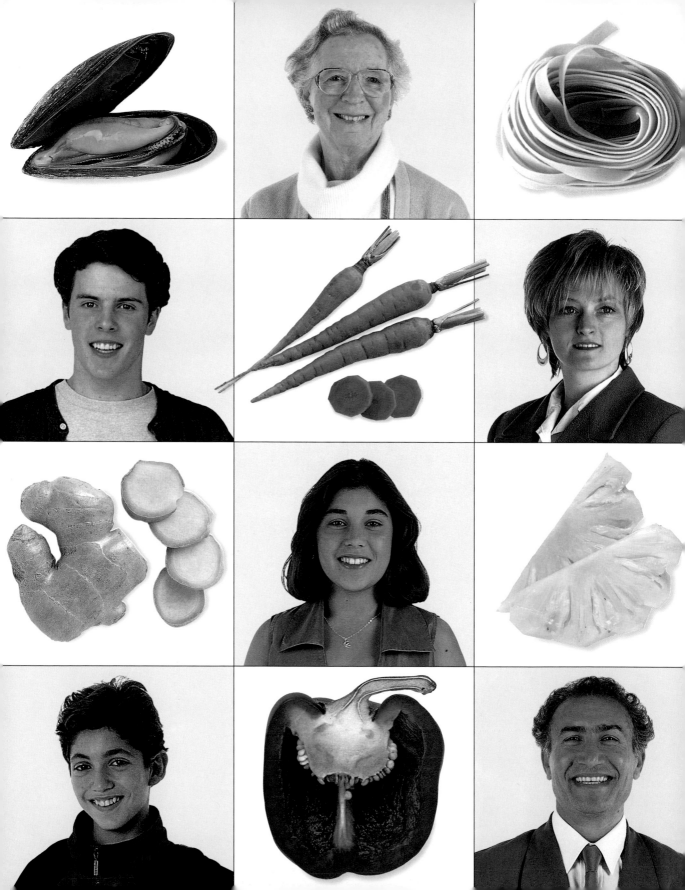

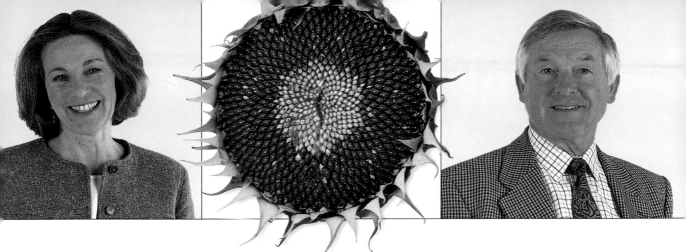

IMPROVING
YOUR HEALTH

A practical guide showing which foods to eat to help

prevent or relieve a wide range of common health problems, from

skin complaints to gallstones. Note: Whatever the condition,

eating a balanced diet is the main step to staying well, see pp. 12–13.

The information in this book is not given as medical advice, which should be sought for any worrying or persistent symptoms.

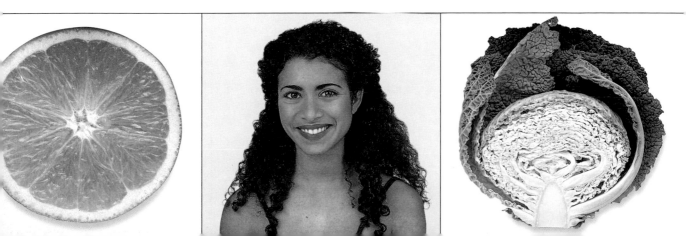

RESPIRATORY SYSTEM

INFLAMMATION OF THE mucous lining and the production of extra mucus are part of the body's reaction to infection and irritant substances. Eating more of certain foods can help the body's defenses fight infection and aid the relief of symptoms such as a sore throat, blocked nose, and painful sinuses. Certain foods may be able to help asthma by countering bronchial constriction. Some respiratory symptoms are adverse reactions to particular foods.

❖ INFECTIONS ❖

Well-balanced eating is important to your resistance to illness: shortage of any one of the essential nutrients will reduce your defensive ability.

GENERAL ADVICE

• *Eat plenty of foods containing key nutrients for resistance to infection, see The Body's Defenses, p. 89.*
• *Give up smoking.*

COLDS & FLU

Colds and flu are mainly viral infections. The body's reaction to the cold virus inflames the mucous lining of the nose and throat, causing a blocked or runny nose and a sore throat. Flu symptoms are variable, and may include fever, aches, pains, and sickness. A cough is the body's attempt to remove mucus or irritants from the airways.
• Fever is a natural part of the body's defenses, so do not suppress it unless it is very high. Drink plenty of fluids to replace those lost in sweating.
• Inhale steam for at least 4 minutes twice a day: it is one of the best proven ways to fight respiratory infection.

HELPFUL FOODS

• *Shellfish, pumpkin seeds, lean meat, liver, and dairy foods* are rich in zinc, which can reduce the length of some colds.
• *Black currants, green leafy vegetables, red peppers, and citrus fruits* are rich in vitamin C. A good supply may help kill the bacteria present in some respiratory illnesses. It has not been proved that large doses of vitamin C shorten or relieve colds.

• *Garlic, watercress, and onion* are anti-infective and are traditionally used for respiratory complaints. Watercress and onion can also help relieve bronchial congestion, and garlic has antiviral effects.
• *Green tea* has countered the flu virus in laboratory tests and, in Asia, has long been used for fever.
• *Ginger and chili peppers* can help relieve congested airways and associated headache by stimulating the circulation and thinning mucus so it is disposed of more quickly. Ginger dries up phlegm and also helps the body cough it up.
• *Ginger, fennel, and chili peppers* have warming, antispasmodic, and settling effects that can help gastric symptoms.
• *Honey* can soothe a sore throat and help voice loss.
• *Crushed fennel seeds* are traditionally used for wheeziness and dry coughs. For a warming, relaxing effect, eat them, make them into a tea, or mix them with hot water and inhale the steam.

❖ ASTHMA & ❖ ALLERGIES

Strictly speaking, "allergy" refers only to an overreaction to a protein by the immune system. Nonallergic adverse reactions can be just as real. Many substances entering the body through the mouth, skin, or by inhalation can cause reactions, and are thought to be responsible for most cases of asthma.

GENERAL ADVICE

• *Identify substances that cause the reaction and try to avoid them. To detect possible food culprits, see p. 79.*

ASTHMA

Asthma attacks can be triggered by many irritants. Emotion or stress can play a major part. Bronchial passages become inflamed, making breathing difficult, with wheeziness and coughing.
• Brisk exercise, yoga, and breathing exercises can help avert attacks.

HELPFUL FOODS

• *Onion* may help prevent some asthma attacks, perhaps because it counters bronchial constriction.
• *Tea* contains a relative of caffeine called theophylline, which has a mild bronchodilating effect. It has been used in a concentrated form to treat asthma attacks.

ALLERGIES

Respiratory symptoms such as excess mucus, congested sinuses, and hay fever (allergic rhinitis) are often caused by reactions to substances in food, air, or the products we encounter. Some adverse reactions occur exclusively at times of illness, low resistance, or stress. The only proven treatment for such adverse reactions is to avoid the cause. Some alternative practitioners claim to be able to make people less sensitive to the substances that irritate them. This has not been proved, although honey has been traditionally used in this way.

HELPFUL FOODS

• *Honey containing pollen, either unfiltered cold-pressed liquid honey or honeycomb,* has traditionally been used to desensitize hay fever sufferers, see p. 65.

EYES & MOUTH

EYESIGHT AND MOUTH PROBLEMS tend to be accepted as inevitable, especially as people get older, but many can be avoided or reduced by eating well. Preventive care of the eyes and mouth is most effective when started young. The health of the mouth is especially dependent on healthy eating, and vice versa: poor dental health or dentures make eating fresh vegetables and fruits much more difficult, prejudicing overall well-being and resistance to infection.

❖ EYES ❖

The most common minor eye disorders are the result of inflammation or infection, but they can also be a sign of wider problems or a side effect of drugs. Twitching eyelids are usually a sign of nervousness, see p. 93, or tiredness.

GENERAL ADVICE

• *Seek emergency advice for sudden inflammation, eye pressure, floaters, or blurred vision, which can be symptoms of glaucoma or detached retina.*
• *Identify and avoid eye irritants such as makeup and swimming pool chlorine.*
• *Have regular eye tests.*

DETERIORATING EYESIGHT

Although eyesight naturally declines with age, deterioration can be related to poor circulation, in which food plays a major part. See also Circulation, p. 82.

HELPFUL FOODS

Black currants, blueberries, bilberries, citrus fruits, cranberries, green leafy vegetables, and red peppers are rich in flavonoids or vitamin C. These help maintain efficient circulation and the strength of small capillary blood vessels.
Sunflower seeds, sweet potatoes, walnuts, and almonds contain vitamin E and essential fatty acids, which discourage inflammation and help the circulation.

STIES & CONJUNCTIVITIS

These infections are more likely to occur if poor nutrition reduces resistance.

• Wash your hands before rubbing eyes or touching contact lenses.

HELPFUL FOODS

Foods that support the immune system, p. 89, help the body counter infection.

CATARACTS & MACULAR DEGENERATION

Cataract, a clouding of the eye lens, and degeneration of the macula (the part of the retina involved in fine vision) are the main causes of loss of sight in elderly people in developed countries. Recent research shows a strong link between eating habits early in life and macular degeneration and cataracts.

HELPFUL FOODS

• *Green leafy vegetables, sunflower seeds, sweet potatoes, winter squash, apricots, carrots, black currants, and citrus fruits* are rich in the antioxidants beta-carotene and vitamins C and E. Although these eye conditions involve many factors, there is strong evidence that people who eat plenty of foods rich in these antioxidants are less at risk.

❖ MOUTH ❖

Dental hygiene is valuable, but it cannot maintain the health of the mouth without good eating habits.

DENTAL CARIES

Sugar is the main cause of dental caries. The number of times sugar is eaten is more important than the quantity, and sugar eaten with a meal causes less decay than when it is eaten alone.

• Brush teeth and remove food debris after eating, especially after sugary foods.
• Have regular dental checkups and get prompt treatment for broken fillings in which food can get trapped.
• Saliva helps counter bacteria and can be encouraged by chewing well.

HELPFUL FOODS

• *Cheese,* eaten as a small cube at the end of a meal, can reduce the risk of decay and possibly help remineralization.
• *Tea* is rich in fluoride, which, in low-fluoride areas, helps to reduce tooth decay.

GUM DISEASE (GINGIVITIS)

Teeth are as readily lost through gum disease as through dental caries. Infection arises from bacteria living on food particles around the teeth.
• Follow advice for Dental Caries, *above.*

HELPFUL FOODS

• *Green leafy vegetables, citrus fruits, black currants, and red peppers* are rich in vitamin C and flavonoids, needed to prevent bleeding and spongy gums and to prevent teeth from becoming loose.

COLD SORES

These are caused by the *herpes simplex* virus. Once you have caught the virus it remains for life, although outbreaks may occur only in times of stress.
• The virus is highly contagious: avoid contact with anyone with a cold sore.

HELPFUL FOODS

• *Oysters, lean meat, pumpkin seeds, and milk products* are zinc-rich foods that may bring relief.

DIGESTIVE SYSTEM

 DIGESTIVE DISORDERS ARE OFTEN overlooked as minor, but they are a common cause of discomfort. They can also be a warning that changes in lifestyle are needed to avoid more serious illnesses: heartburn can lead to ulcers; indigestion after fatty food to gallbladder disease. Our digestive health also affects how well we absorb nutrients from food, for overall well-being. Heredity makes some people more vulnerable to digestive disorders than others, but lifestyle also plays an important part. Healthier eating habits are the main step in preventing and relieving most digestive disorders.

❖ DIGESTIVE ❖ DISORDERS

Eating habits involving a high intake of fat, heavy meals, a lack of fiber, too much coffee and alcohol, too many carbonated beverages, and eating when not hungry are likely, in time, to cause digestive problems for most people. The body's reaction to stress or an adverse reaction to a food may also affect the digestive system.

GENERAL ADVICE

• *Make sensible eating a priority, especially if digestive disorders are common in your family.*
• *Eat food slowly and chew well.*
• *Pay attention to what your body wants you to eat, and never eat something you do not want.*
• *Avoid excessive amounts of alcohol, although a little may help.*
• *Improve stress resistance with techniques such as yoga or meditation.*
• *Physical activity can help combat stress and is known to improve mood.*

CONSTIPATION

Although increasing the amount of cereal fiber eaten is a proven way to treat constipation, it is important to address other causes such as lack of fluid, inactivity, delaying the urge to defecate, and habitual use of laxatives or antacids.
• Build up the amount of fiber you eat over several weeks. A sudden rise can lead to flatulence and bloating.
• Never ignore the need to go to the toilet.

HELPFUL FOODS

• *Whole-grain bread, pasta, and cereals* are rich in fiber. Gradually increase intake to about 6–7 slices of whole-grain bread a day, or 3–4 slices of bread and 1¾ oz (50g) whole-grain cereals.
• *Vegetables and fruits, especially apples, dried apricots, and less ripe bananas* discourage constipation and provide fluid. Build up to eating about 14oz (400g) a day.
• *Linseed* is a gentle laxative. Take 1 heaping tablespoon a day with 5fl oz (150ml) fluid until constipation is resolved.
• *Yogurt with active cultures and raw sauerkraut* can help foster the bacteria that provide most of the bulk in stools.

DIVERTICULAR DISEASE

Low-fiber eating may result in "blow outs" in the walls of the intestines, caused by the pressure of muscles straining to move small stools along. Waste lodging in these pockets can become infected, causing acute pain and inflammation.

HELPFUL FOODS

• *Unrefined cereal grains* rich in insoluble fiber increase stool bulk. Choose a variety of whole-wheat bread made with extra, coarse-textured bran.

FLATULENCE

The production of some gas is a natural part of digestion. Excess gas can be caused by heavy meals, antacids, and swallowing air – for example, while talking. It may also be caused by excessive amounts of the common yeast *Candida albicans*, see p. 87.
• Eat slowly and do not gulp drinks.

HELPFUL FOODS

• *Fennel root and seeds, dill, angelica (archangelica variety), cinnamon, caraway, and cardamom* help prevent and relieve flatulence by warming and relaxing the digestive tract. Yogurt containing active *Lb. acidophilus* cultures can counter gas caused by *Candida albicans* and fosters bacteria that can help digestion.

DIARRHEA & VOMITING

Both diarrhea and vomiting are evidence of the body ridding itself of harmful substances, such as drugs or a bacteria or virus, and should not be suppressed in adults for the first 36 hours.
• Keep warm and drink plenty of fluid to prevent dehydration.
• Do not eat unless you want to.

HELPFUL FOODS

• *Ginger* can help prevent nausea and colicky spasms.
• *Garlic, live yogurt, black currants, cold-pressed honey, apples, and ripe bananas* are traditional treatments for diarrhea. Eat them as soon as possible after the attack.
• *Chili peppers and watercress* encourage the production of sterilizing digestive acid and guard against the recurrence of diarrhea and vomiting.
• *Yogurt with active cultures and raw sauerkraut* can help restore healthy gut flora in the intestines during recovery.

• *Wheat germ and chicken liver* help restore B vitamins, which can be depleted by an attack of diarrhea.

INDIGESTION

Indigestion has a variety of causes, including stress, eating too much or too quickly, and eating fatty or spicy foods.
• Eat less fat, which puts extra strain on the digestive system.
• Improving the circulation can help, see Circulation, pp. 82–5.

HELPFUL FOODS

• *Chili peppers (if tolerated) and watercress* encourage digestive juices.
• *Pineapple* can help protein digestion.
• *Linseed and oats* are rich in mucilage, which soothes the digestive tract.
• *Ginger and cinnamon* have a warming effect and help relieve gut spasms.
• *Asparagus* can help relieve sluggish digestion by speeding the emptying of the stomach.

GASTROENTERITIS

Bacteria, a virus, or toxins from the resulting food poisoning can all cause inflammation of the digestive tract, with cramps, vomiting, fever, or diarrhea. The best defense is good food hygiene. See also Diarrhea & Vomiting, p. 78.

HELPFUL FOODS

• *Garlic, yogurt with active cultures, bilberries, cranberries, and cold-pressed honey* have shown antibacterial action.

PEPTIC ULCERS

Ulcers are irritated or raw patches in the walls of the digestive tract, caused either by excess acid or by damage to the mucous lining that normally protects the walls from the acid. Susceptibility to ulcers can be hereditary, and although stress is unlikely to cause an ulcer it can worsen an existing one. Infection with *Helicobacter pylori* and adverse reactions to foods can also be causes.
• Milky, low-fiber diets are not effective, and too much milk can encourage acid production.
• Avoid drugs such as aspirin and other nonsteroidal anti-inflammatory drugs that attack the mucous lining.
• Avoid alcohol, caffeine, and heavy meals, which overstimulate acid production.

• Avoid the regular use of antacids, which can cause "rebound" rise in acid.
• Give up smoking. Tobacco slows the healing of ulcers.

HELPFUL FOODS

• *Raw cabbage and green plantains (cooked)* can help ulcers heal and discourage recurrence.
• *Cold-pressed manuka honey and yogurt with active* Lb. acidophilus *cultures* counter **Helicobacter pylori** bacteria.
• *Shellfish, pumpkin seeds, and other zinc-rich foods* help ensure adequate zinc, needed for wound-healing.
• *Oats, legumes, apples, linseed, sunflower seeds, black currants, black raspberries, and raspberries* are high in soluble fiber, which may help discourage ulcer recurrence. Mucilage-rich oats and linseed help protect the mucous lining of the digestive tract from irritation.

GALLSTONES

Common among those eating Western-style diets, gallstones are crystals of cholesterol or calcium, or both. They form when the body produces more cholesterol than usual in its digestive bile, or when the bile is too high in calcium. Gallstones can block the exit of bile to the intestine. Fat is not digested and inflammation results, causing nausea, indigestion, pain, and loss of fat-soluble vitamins. Vegetarians are 50% less likely to suffer from gallstones than those who eat meat.
• Limit fats and alcohol, although a little alcohol is beneficial.
• Eat plenty of fruits and vegetables.
• Watch your weight. There is a strong link between gallstones and excess weight in women under 50, and in men with large paunches.
• Avoid constipation, p. 78, which increases the risk of gallstones.

HELPFUL FOODS

• *Artichokes and bitter greens such as radicchio and dandelion leaves* stimulate bile production, which helps dilute cholesterol and calcium. Artichoke has been shown to help relieve gallbladder discomfort and to aid liver health.
• *Oats, legumes, vegetables, and fruits* are rich in soluble fiber, which helps limit the rise in blood sugar after eating. High blood sugar levels tend to raise bile cholesterol. Soluble fiber can also cause cholesterol excretion.

DETECTING FOODS THAT DO NOT AGREE ❖ WITH YOU ❖

Warning
"Exclusion diets," where the diet is reduced to only 2 or 3 foods and items are reintroduced gradually, should be carried out only with professional supervision.

Excluding a food from your diet is the only reliable method of determining whether it is to blame for your health disorder. Choose one type of food at a time, and completely exclude all forms of it from your diet for about 2–3 weeks. This should be long enough to show whether the food is worth avoiding.

• Always eat a replacement food to supply similar nutrients. For example, dairy foods supply an important share of calcium, zinc, and vitamin B2. If you exclude them, you can replace the calcium by eating tofu, almonds, canned sardines including the bones, and green leafy vegetables. You can replace the zinc with shellfish, lean meat, or pumpkin seeds; and the vitamin B2 with liver, wheat germ, almonds, or pumpkin seeds.
• Although some food additives can cause reactions in certain people, an adverse reaction is much more likely from nutritious everyday foods. The foods thought most likely to cause adverse reactions are milk, eggs, wheat, fish, shellfish, soy, peanuts and other nuts, pork, tenderized meats, chocolate, coffee, tea, and citrus fruits.
• The above list includes several foods used in weaning. Giving solids or cow's milk to babies when they are too young to cope with them is thought to be a factor in the development of some adverse reactions.
• The food additives most often linked with adverse reactions are synthetic colors, the benzoate, sulfur, and gallate preservatives, and glutamate flavor enhancers.
• Intolerance to a food may be part of a temporary health condition: if you have an adverse reaction to a food it might not be permanent. It is therefore worth trying excluded foods again (with the exception of nuts and peanuts) after 6 months or a year.

BONES & JOINTS

BONE AND JOINT DISORDERS are widely regarded as wear-and-tear illnesses of age, but they are more often the cumulative results of disorders of body chemistry in which food and lifestyle play a major part. The reliance of orthodox treatment on drugs with substantial side effects gives every incentive to try more natural methods to gain relief. Diet is increasingly recognized as having an important role in both prevention and relief.

❖ BONES ❖

Our bones continually renew and repair themselves, making their care a lifelong matter. Although skeletal development peaks in teenagers, bone density increases until around the age of 40. Limiting bone loss as we age is important to protect freedom of movement and thereby safeguard independence. Although heredity plays a part in bone health, many factors are under our own control.

GENERAL ADVICE

• *A good intake of calcium is important, particularly in childhood when needs are highest, but there is no benefit in exceeding the recommended amount, see p. 150. Excess calcium is known to interfere with the absorption of iron and can encourage kidney stones in people prone to them.*
• *Eating well in general is as important as adequate calcium intake to ensure the growth and maintenance of strong, dense bones, see the Basic Healthy Diet, pp. 12–13.*
• *Avoid too much salt, protein, sugar, and too many carbonated beverages with phosphoric acid, all of which cause more calcium to be excreted.*
• *Vitamin D is needed for calcium absorption. Help the body manufacture vitamin D by spending time outside in sunlight with exposed arms and legs.*
• *Look after your kidneys, see p. 92, where vitamin D is activated.*

OSTEOPOROSIS

"Osteoporosis" means porous bones. In this condition, large amounts of minerals are lost from the bones, leaving them prone to fracture and poor healing. The absorption of calcium into the bones is stimulated by the sex hormones. Osteoporosis generally appears earlier in women because the production of sex hormones starts declining earlier, at menopause. Some women make use of hormone replacement therapy (HRT), which reduces the loss of bone minerals. The effects are not permanent, however, unless it is taken for the rest of their lives. Both sexes are equally affected by the other factors involved in osteoporosis, and can benefit from improving their lifestyle and diet.
• Get daily weight-bearing exercise, such as walking. This is the most effective way to avoid, slow, and reverse bone loss. Carrying even a few pounds of extra weight, such as a bag of groceries, increases this benefit.
• Avoid smoking and alcohol, both of which accelerate bone density loss.

HELPFUL FOODS

• *Milk, yogurt, and hard cheese* are the richest sources of calcium and are easily absorbed. Lack of calcium in youth may mean bones do not reach their density potential, but lack of calcium after 40 is not a major factor in osteoporosis. Eating more than the recommended levels of calcium in food or supplements has not been proved to help postmenopausal bone strength.
• *Tofu, fish such as canned sardines or whitebait, both eaten with their bones, almonds, and green leafy vegetables, especially broccoli and watercress,* are the best nondairy sources of calcium.

• *Oily fish* is the main food source of vitamin D, which is needed for calcium absorption.
• *Soy protein foods such as tofu, soybeans, soy flour, and soy milk* contain phytoestrogens. (Note: not soybean oil; TVP is not a reliable source.) In a recent study, postmenopausal women who ate 1½ oz (45g) of soy grits (chopped beans) a day for 12 weeks had improved lumbar spine density compared with a control group.

❖ JOINTS & MUSCLES ❖

The joints are encased in smooth cartilage and are padded and lubricated by synovial membrane and fluid. They work with the surrounding network of ligaments and muscles to enable smooth movement. The joints are vulnerable to wear and tear, especially if the muscles that share their weight load are weak or overstrained. They are also affected by disorders of the metabolism, which can be related to what we eat.

GENERAL ADVICE

• *Maintain muscle tone with moderate exercise to protect joints from strain.*
• *Avoid becoming overweight, which strains the joints.*
• *Eat a well-balanced diet, see pp. 12–13, to help the efficiency of the liver, adrenal glands, and kidneys. These regulate the content of body fluids, which in turn affect the health of the joints.*

GOUT

The tendency to gout is strongly hereditary, but it can be reduced by careful eating habits among those who know they are at risk: particularly overweight men who have close relatives with gout. Joint pain and swelling are caused when the body has an excess of uric acid, which is the waste product of purines mainly found in protein foods. The acid forms crystals that are deposited in the joints, kidneys, and other tissues. Most sufferers produce more uric acid than normal, while a smaller number cannot dispose of uric acid normally.
• Lose weight if needed, but gradually. Near-fasting can trigger an attack.
• Avoid alcohol, which increases uric acid production.
• Try not to take diuretic drugs, which raise the blood level of uric acid.
• Avoid foods high in purines: liver, shellfish, kidneys, game, yeast, sardines; and to some extent asparagus, spinach, cauliflower, mushrooms, and peas.

HELPFUL FOODS

• *Cherries:* red, black, fresh, or canned, have relieved gout in several cases, when at least 15–25 (8oz or 225g) were eaten per day.
• *Arthritis diet, right,* excluding the high-purine foods, *above,* may help.

ARTHRITIS & RHEUMATISM

One of mankind's most common health problems, arthritis has many different forms, causing different patterns of swelling and pain in joints. Often bracketed with muscular pain under the general name of rheumatism, there are 2 main types. In osteoarthritis, joint cartilage breaks down or hardens and bones distort, developing lumps and spurs. In rheumatoid arthritis, joints are inflamed, causing pain, fever, and stiffness. There has been relatively little exploration of the contribution of food to prevention, but there is increasing evidence that diet can be a useful treatment.

GENERAL ADVICE

• Maintain a healthy weight.
• Tension and stress play a part, so tackle them with rest, light exercise, and stress-management techniques such as meditation or gentle yoga.

❖ ARTHRITIS DIET ❖

Arthritis diets are based on two ideas. One is that some forms of arthritis are caused or aggravated by years of unbalanced eating and stress. Combined with stress management, a vegetarian diet of mainly vegetables, unrefined carbohydrates, nuts, and seeds may produce relief after several months. The other idea is that some cases of rheumatoid arthritis may be an adverse reaction to particular foods, which must be avoided. The eating plan below is partly based on the diet used for arthritis by Dr. John Hunter's clinic at Addenbrooke's Hospital, Cambridge, UK.

.... *Caution* ....
Do not reduce any medication.

• For 4 weeks, avoid completely: tea, coffee, chocolate, sugar, alcohol, cows' milk products, meat (except for poultry), shellfish (except for New Zealand green-lipped mussels), sardines, citrus fruits, pickled or smoked food, wheat, rye, barley, soy products such as tofu, peanuts, and eggs.
• Avoid all foods with added sugar.
• Reduce salt and fat as much as possible apart from 1–1¾ oz (25–50g) nuts or seeds a day and the same amount of oil or all-vegetable margarine a day.
• Base meals on vegetables, fruits, nuts, seeds, and unrefined cereal grains, with small servings of higher protein foods.
• After 4 weeks:
Reintroduce 1 food every 4 days, and observe your reaction. Introduce staples such as milk, wheat, meat, and eggs first. Any food that causes an adverse reaction can be excluded again.

HELPFUL FOODS

• *Oily fish* has helped rheumatoid arthritis in trials. Eat about 1lb 9oz (700g) a week.
• *Fresh ginger,* when 1¾ oz (50g) cooked or ¼ oz (5g) raw a day was eaten, gave some relief to most sufferers of osteo- or rheumatoid arthritis in Danish trials.
• *Raw pineapple and chili peppers* have shown some anti-inflammatory action.

• *Green-lipped mussels* are an unproved but popular remedy in extract form.
• *Apples, asparagus, black currants, celery, and parsley* have traditionally been used for arthritis relief.

OPTIONAL SUPPLEMENTS

These have all produced some relief of symptoms in at least 1 clinical trial.
• *Vitamin E:* take 400mg a day.
• *Vitamin C:* take 1g 4 times a day, reducing after relief to 500mg daily.
• *Bromelain enzymes:* take 125–400mg 3 times daily.
• *Pantothenic acid* (for rheumatoid arthritis): take 500mg a day for 2 days; 1g daily for 3 days; 1,500mg daily for 4 days; then 200mg a day for 2 months or until pain is relieved. Then reduce to the minimum needed to maintain relief.

TYPICAL MENU

Breakfast
• Oatmeal or oat muesli, fresh or soaked dried fruit, herb tea, or coffee substitute

Snacks
• Fresh or dried fruit; sunflower and pumpkin seeds

Light Meals
• Waldorf Salad, p. 110, dressed with unrefined sunflower oil

• Baked sweet or ordinary potato with all-vegetable margarine *or* a legume dish, for example, Lima Beans with Sage & Garlic, p. 125, Dhal, p. 127, or Low-Fat Hummus, p. 140

Main Meals
• Vegetable Chowder, p. 103
Grilled salmon *or* Broccoli Stir-Fry, p. 121, served with brown rice or kasha, and green leafy vegetables
Baked sweet apple with chopped dates *or* fresh pineapple

Drinks
• Unlimited herb tea and coffee substitutes; 1 glass per day of unsweetened apple or grape juice; use oat or rice "milk" if desired

Seasonings
• Parsley, celery seeds, garlic, ginger, chili peppers, and onion

CIRCULATION & HEART HEALTH

IMPROVING THE EFFICIENCY of the circulation is one of the most rewarding effects of eating for health. Many aspects of health, from energy to eyesight, are affected by the supply of oxygen and nourishment to the cells. Impaired circulation is linked to conditions ranging from heart disease and stroke to varicose veins and poor resistance to infection. What we eat affects the circulation by helping or hindering the heart and by influencing the elasticity of blood vessels, the ability of the blood to carry oxygen, and its tendency to form clots.

CIRCULATION ❖ HEALTH ❖

Although circulation health is to some extent hereditary, it is also closely connected to living habits. People who eat a Western-style diet tend to accumulate fatty plaque on the walls of their arteries, leading to atherosclerosis (narrowing and hardening of the arteries). This damages the circulation, bringing the risk of coronary heart disease, stroke, and poor peripheral circulation with many related disorders such as varicose veins, cramps, and a reduced supply of oxygen to the brain. Narrowed arteries raise blood pressure, making the heart work harder, and fatty plaque is rich in cholesterol, so measuring blood pressure and blood cholesterol can show the extent of atherosclerosis.

Both high blood pressure and high cholesterol levels can be radically improved by changes in eating habits. It is best to start taking steps in childhood, but changes later in life help too: for example, studies of people who have survived a heart attack show that those who change their diet can dramatically improve their chances of surviving future heart attacks.

Good circulation also depends on blood health. Two common problems are blood that forms clots too readily, leading to risk of blocked blood vessels, and iron deficiency, which reduces the oxygen-carrying ability of the blood.

GENERAL ADVICE

• *Eat less fat, especially saturated fat, which, in excess, encourages both deposits of fatty plaque in the arteries, see High Blood Cholesterol, p. 83, and excessive blood clotting.*
• *Stop smoking and avoid excess alcohol: both encourage hardening of the arteries.*
• *Get brisk exercise daily, maintain good posture, and breathe deeply.*

HEART DISEASE & STROKE

Coronary heart disease occurs when the arteries carrying oxygen-bearing blood to the heart become so narrow that the supply is reduced. A complete blockage, due to a blood clot forming in the artery wall or plaque breaking away frrom the wall, will precipitate a heart attack or, if it occurs in an artery supplying the brain, a stroke. Key risk factors for both heart disease and stroke are high blood pressure, high blood-clotting factors, and a low intake of foods rich in the antioxidants vitamin E, beta-carotene, and, to a lesser extent, vitamin C. In addition, high blood cholesterol means a higher risk of a heart attack. The blood's ability to clot is essential to heal wounds. However, eating a high level of fat, particularly saturated fat, as well as smoking, taking oral contraceptives, and being overweight, especially around the waist, can encourage the blood to clot too readily in the veins or arteries.
• Follow General Advice for Circulation Health, *above.*
• Take steps to avoid or reduce raised blood cholesterol and blood pressure.
• Try to maintain a healthy weight, as obesity sharply increases stroke and heart disease risk. Keep your Body Mass Index (BMI) to 25 or under, see p. 87.
• Monitor your alcohol intake. A small amount of any alcohol, up to 3½ fl oz (100ml) a week, is linked to a halved risk of stroke, probably because it dilates the blood vessels. This is equivalent to about 12 x ¾ fl oz (20ml) measures of whiskey or 5–6 x 5fl oz (150ml) glasses of red wine. A lower risk of heart disease is linked to 1–3 glasses of red wine daily, a benefit thought to be due to its alcohol and flavonoid content. However, more than these amounts increases the risk of stroke and coronary heart disease.

HELPFUL FOODS

• *Oily fish such as sardines, salmon, and mackerel* contain the omega-3 fatty acid eicosapentaenoic acid (EPA), which discourages the clotting tendency of the blood. Little research is available, but in theory the body can make EPA from alpha-linolenic acid found in foods such as linseed, wheat germ, and walnuts. However, oily fish is the best proven source of this nutrient. Eat some at least twice a week.
• *Sunflower products, almonds, sweet potatoes, and wheat germ* are rich in vitamin E, the antioxidant most strongly linked with a lower risk of angina and heart attack. The typical Western-style diet provides around 10mg, and research evidence suggests it is worthwhile to aim for at least 40mg a day.
• *Green leafy vegetables, carrots, apricots, winter squash, orange-fleshed sweet potatoes, and red peppers* are outstanding sources of beta-carotene. In ample amounts from food, this is linked to a lower risk of

stroke and, for smokers and former smokers, a lowered risk of heart disease.
• *Black currants, strawberries, citrus fruits, red peppers, and green leafy vegetables such as watercress* are very rich in antioxidant vitamin C, which is needed daily.
• *Onions, tea, red wine, and apples* are the main sources of the flavonoid quercetin, which has recently been linked to a lower risk of heart disease and stroke. The protective potential may be due to an antioxidant action.
• *Onions, garlic, chili peppers, ginger, pineapple, and tea* discourage blood clotting. Onions, garlic, and chili peppers can also help blood flow more freely by dilating the blood vessels.

HIGH BLOOD PRESSURE

High blood pressure is one of the main indications of coronary heart disease and stroke risk.
• Follow General Advice for Circulation Health, p. 82.
• Eat less salt, which is mainly sodium and, in excess, raises blood pressure in many people. Buy less processed food: at least two-thirds of the salt we eat has already been added by manufacturers.

HELPFUL FOODS

• *Dried apricots, potatoes, sweet potatoes, black currants, celery, fennel, green leafy vegetables, parsley, artichokes, and legumes* are all high in potassium, which helps regulate blood pressure by enabling the body to dispose of more sodium.
• *Garlic and oats* can help reduce raised blood pressure.
• *Lemon juice, fresh herbs, spices, small amounts of honey, and vinegar* may be used to flavor food instead of salt.

HIGH BLOOD CHOLESTEROL

High overall levels of blood cholesterol are a danger sign, warning of higher risk of coronary heart disease. However, the cholesterol in the blood includes some "good" high density lipoprotein (HDL), which helps move cholesterol to the liver for disposal. Lowering cholesterol healthily means maintaining or raising HDL while reducing "bad" low density lipoprotein (LDL) cholesterol, which contributes to atherosclerosis, see Circulation Health, p. 82.
• Follow General Advice for Circulation Health, p. 82.
• Reduce your intake of saturated and

trans fatty acids to about 10% of calories in total (typically about 20g a day for women and 22g for men). Above this quantity, both increase levels of cholesterol in the blood and encourage clotting. Saturated and trans fatty acids (often labeled on packaged foods as "hydrogenated") are the main fats in cheese, meat, cookies, cakes, pastry, chocolate, whole-milk products, and any fat that is solid at room temperature.

HELPFUL FOODS

• *Artichokes, onion, and 1–2 cloves of garlic a day* can help lower blood cholesterol, although it is not known why.
• *Walnuts, sunflower seeds, almonds, pumpkin seeds, linseed, wheat germ, and soybeans* all provide linoleic acid, the essential fatty acid that lowers total cholesterol and, to some extent, reduces the tendency of the blood to form harmful clots. Eat small regular amounts: too much linoleic acid will lower HDL as well as LDL cholesterol.
• *Oats, legumes, apples, dried and citrus fruits, and peas* are rich in soluble fiber, which reduces the amount of LDL cholesterol entering the bloodstream. Soluble fiber needs a low-fat diet to work well. Oats can also lower raised blood pressure.

❖ HEALTHY EATING PLAN ❖

These sample menus show how foods that help heart health and help reduce the risk of stroke can fit into an enjoyable, low-fat style of eating.

General
• Use low-fat sunflower margarine, skim milk, and low-fat salad dressings.

Breakfasts
• Oatmeal with added oat bran and wheat germ; an orange or a grapefruit

• Whole-wheat toast with low-fat sunflower margarine and black currant jam or jelly

• Real Muesli, p. 131, with wheat germ and sunflower seeds; an orange

• Baked beans on whole-grain toast; toast with low-fat sunflower margarine and honey

• Poached egg on whole-wheat toast; an orange or a grapefruit

Snacks
• Oat Bran Muffins, p. 137; apples; sunflower seeds; dried apricots; bananas; almonds; carrots

Light Meals
• Lentil soup; Waldorf Salad, p. 110
• Baked sweet potato with Slaw Salad, p.112

• Carrot & Cilantro Soup, p. 100; celery and walnut sandwich

• Munkazina Salad, p. 109; Honey & Lemon Cheesecake, p. 131

• Salmon sandwich with Sunflower Green Salad, p. 112

• Low-Fat Hummus, p. 140, with pita bread and Slaw Salad, p. 112

Main Meals
• Swiss Onion Soup, p. 102
Grilled salmon with Pineapple Salsa, p. 138, with Sweet Potato Chips, p. 126, and green beans or peas
Cranberry & Apricot Compote, p. 132

• Dill Marinated Herrings, p. 106, with oatcakes
Broccoli Stir-Fry, p. 121, with chili sauce and brown rice with sunflower seeds
Fresh pineapple

• Lima Beans with Sage & Garlic, p. 125
Forty-Clove Garlic Chicken, p. 117, with red cabbage and watercress salad
Baked Ginger Bananas, p. 129

• Swiss Onion Soup, p. 102
Celery Amandine, p. 120, with baked sweet potato
Kissel, p. 133, made with black currants

• Warm Walnut Dip with Grilled Vegetables, p. 105
Falafel, p. 123, and Low-Fat Hummus, p. 140, with whole-wheat pita
Apricot Almond Fool, p. 130

• Arame, Broccoli & Walnut Salad, p. 110
Greek Fish Stew made with oily fish, p. 115; Spiced Winter Squash, p. 125
Sunflower, Apple & Apricot Crumble, p. 133

❖ OTHER CIRCULATION ❖ & BLOOD DISORDERS

Eating more foods to improve the circulation not only helps reduce the risk of stroke and heart disease, but also can benefit a wide range of lesser, but nevertheless debilitating health problems, from low energy levels and dizziness to cold feet and easy bruising.

GENERAL ADVICE

• *Follow General Advice for Circulation Health, p. 82.*

FLUID RETENTION

In good health, the body has the ability to maintain a precise fluid balance. Retaining too much fluid not only is uncomfortable, but also can be an indication of an underlying condition, such as heart disease or high blood pressure, pp. 82–3, enlarged prostate, p. 93, or premenstrual syndrome, p. 86. Fluid retention can also be a side effect of steroid drugs. Some specialists believe that fluid retention can be the result of a food allergy, p. 79.
• Avoid salty foods. Excess sodium puts a strain on the kidneys, and most Western-style diets contain too much sodium-based salt.

HELPFUL FOODS

• *Dried apricots, artichokes, bananas, black currants, celery, citrus fruits, fennel, green leafy vegetables, parsley, potatoes, and legumes* are rich in potassium, which the kidneys need to excrete excess sodium. If you are prescribed diuretic drugs, it is particularly important to eat plenty of these foods to restore potassium levels.
• *Asparagus, artichokes, black currants, celery, dandelion leaves, and parsley* increase urine output and therefore can help some cases of fluid retention.

VARICOSE VEINS & HEMORRHOIDS

The muscular action of the calves and thighs pumps deoxygenated blood upward on its return journey to the heart. The veins in the legs have one-way valves to prevent blood from flowing backward under the force of gravity. If the valves weaken, blood collects in the veins causing them to stretch and bulge. Circulation in the legs worsens, which can lead to painful "heavy" legs and sometimes complications. Varicose veins in the rectum are known as hemorrhoids. Heredity can increase the risk of being prone to varicose veins and hemorrhoids, and other risk factors include poor circulation and obesity.
• Do not restrict the circulation by standing or sitting in one position for long periods or by wearing tight clothing.
• Avoid sitting with the legs crossed.
• Rest with the legs raised above the level of the head.
• Lose weight if necessary and take extra care during pregnancy, when extra weight also puts strain on the circulation in the legs.

HELPFUL FOODS

• *Whole-grain cereals, linseed, dried apricots, and less ripe bananas* combined with plenty of fluid, all prevent constipation, see p. 78, a contributing factor in varicose veins and hemorrhoids.
• *Pineapple, chili peppers, garlic, onion, and ginger* help discourage blood clots. If clots form in the veins, they cause swelling, pain, risk of septicemia, and, if carried to the lungs, risk of a pulmonary embolism.
• *Garlic, ginger, and chili peppers* stimulate the circulation.
• *Green leafy vegetables, bilberries, black currants, citrus fruits, red peppers, and sunflower products* provide a good supply of vitamin C and flavonoids, which help maintain the strength and resilience of blood capillaries.

CHILBLAINS & COLD EXTREMITIES

Chilblains are characterized by itchy red swellings on the extremities that, along with cold hands and feet, are caused by a combination of exposure to cold and poor peripheral circulation. Anemia, p. 85, can reduce the efficiency of the circulation and may be a contributory cause.
• Avoid exposure to cold by wearing warm clothes and shoes that are loose enough to allow good circulation.
• Rub extremities briskly with a rough towel or soft bristle brush toward the heart for 1–2 minutes a day.
• Soak the affected part in hot water for 3 minutes and then in cold water for 1 minute. Repeat 3 times. This stimulates the peripheral circulation.

HELPFUL FOODS

• *Black currants, bilberries, citrus fruits, green leafy vegetables, red peppers, wheat germ, sunflower products, almonds, and sweet potatoes* provide a good supply of vitamins C and E and flavonoids, which are all important for circulation in the small blood vessels.
• *Garlic, ginger, and chili peppers* stimulate circulation and are warming, so eat them freely.

CRAMPS

Sudden spasm in a muscle occurs when the local circulation fails, starving the muscle of oxygen and causing lactic acid, a waste product, to build up. Possible causes include restriction by tight clothing; staying still in one position; anemia; arteries narrowed by heart disease or smoking; lack of calcium or magnesium, which are both needed for muscle contraction; and loss of sodium after heavy sweating.

Caution
Consult a doctor if a cramp is severe or occurs repeatedly. It may be related to heart disease.

ADVICE

• Massage the affected area.
• Drink a mineral-replacing (isotonic) drink, such as fruit juice mixed half and half with water.
• Do not wear tight clothes or shoes.
• Take up some form of aerobic exercise, since it trains the muscles to operate with less oxygen. Do not exercise, however, on a full stomach. Blood will be diverted away from the muscles to help digestion.

HELPFUL FOODS

• *Green leafy vegetables, bilberries, black currants, citrus fruits, red peppers, sunflower products, almonds, wheat germ, and sweet potatoes* provide a good supply of vitamins C and flavonoids, which are important for good circulation.
• *Wheat germ, dried apricots, soybeans, and low-fat yogurt* are rich in magnesium and calcium, a good supply of which is needed for muscle contraction.
• *Garlic, ginger, and chili peppers* stimulate the circulation.

ANEMIA

Anemia occurs when the blood is low in either red blood cells or hemoglobin, meaning that less oxygen reaches the body tissues. The most common causes are a deficiency of nutrients needed to make red blood cells (notably iron, but also folic acid, vitamins B6 and B12, protein, vitamin C, and copper) and loss of blood due to heavy menstruation, bleeding peptic ulcers or hemorrhoids, and regular use of aspirin and many other nonsteroidal pain-relief drugs.

Anemia can result in general weakness, tiredness, and depression, and is surprisingly widespread even in affluent Western countries. Most at risk are teenagers (up to 25% of older girls), pregnant women, and old people. Even mild iron deficiency can reduce energy and resistance to infection, while outright anemia causes dizziness, irritability, palpitations, swollen legs, and lethargy.

Caution

Low levels of hemoglobin should be fully investigated before assuming that they are simply due to iron shortage. Iron supplements should be taken only if blood levels of hemoglobin and ferritin are low. Excess iron can interfere with the absorption of zinc, needed for immune function, and an overload of iron may have an unwanted pro-oxidant effect, see Antioxidants, p. 21.

ADVICE

• Help iron absorption by avoiding a very high calcium intake and by not drinking strong tea with meals (tea roughly halves iron absorption).
• If you may be vulnerable to anemia – for example, if you are taking aspirin regularly or menstruate heavily – you should avoid oat bran and wheat bran (except in whole-wheat bread) because they contain phytic acid, which limits the absorption of iron from food eaten at the same meal.
• Seek treatment for irritable bowel syndrome, as diarrhea prevents nutrients from being absorbed.

HELPFUL FOODS

• *Liver, kidney, oily fish, legumes, dried apricots, black currants, pumpkin seeds, fortified breakfast cereals, green leafy vegetables, wheat germ, and parsley* are top sources of iron and folic acid. It is important to ensure a good supply for hemoglobin production. Vegetarians and vegans should take care to eat enough iron as it is less easily absorbed from plant foods. Women who menstruate heavily, losing a lot of blood, may need more iron than diet alone can supply, but never take supplements without seeking professional advice.
• *Black currants, citrus fruits, strawberries, red peppers, and green leafy vegetables such as watercress* have high levels of vitamin C. Eating a food that is vitamin C-rich (at least 50mg) with every meal can double iron absorption from plant foods.
• *Seaweed* All vegans and a few vegetarians risk slowly developing a shortage of vitamin B12, unless they eat foods fortified with vitamin B12 such as yeast extract and some breakfast cereals, or supplements of the vitamin. Seaweed is almost the only nonanimal source, but absorption is uncertain and substantial amounts must be eaten.
• *Chili peppers, bitter salad greens such as watercress, and artichokes* stimulate digestive juices, which may help people with poor digestion to absorb more of vitamins B12 and B6, folic acid, and iron from food.

❖ CIRCULATION & HEART: QUESTIONS & ANSWERS ❖

• *Do high-cholesterol foods raise the level of cholesterol in the blood?*

Not in the amounts most people eat. It is usually raised by eating excess saturated and trans fatty acids. Many high-cholesterol foods are low in saturated fat, for example, eggs, liver, and shellfish.

• *Can coffee oils (not caffeine) raise blood cholesterol?*

Yes, but only if coffee is made by a method that extracts the oils, for example, boiled by percolation.

• *Are all forms of garlic equally effective at lowering blood cholesterol?*

No. Raw garlic is most effective. Results from dried or puréed garlic and garlic oil capsules have been mixed.

• *Although polyunsaturated fats are better for heart health, can they cause cancer?*

Not if you eat moderate amounts with plenty of foods rich in vitamin E.

• *Is a low-cholesterol level linked to depression?*

It may be in some individuals, but most people who do not eat a Western-style diet have low blood cholesterol rates and do not suffer from depression.

• *Why do some people with low cholesterol and low blood pressure still get heart disease?*

A small number of heart attacks are not caused by coronary heart disease but by various other factors. The heart may become weakened by an infection. Alternatively, inherited levels of a blood constituent called homocysteine may adversely affect the heart. Coronary heart disease, however, is by far the most common risk.

• *Why can some people eat all the wrong foods, smoke 40 cigarettes a day, and still live to be 90?*

Some people inherit a better ability to cope with fat or smoking. There is also evidence that better fetal nutrition and breastfeeding give some protection in later life.

• *Does insoluble fiber, such as wheat bran, lower blood cholesterol?*

No, only soluble fiber can lower cholesterol.

• *Do vegetarians have lower levels of heart disease?*

Yes, but it may be because they eat more fruits and vegetables, or have a more healthy lifestyle in general, rather than because they do not eat meat. Those who eat fish but do not eat meat have even lower levels.

WOMEN'S HEALTH

 IT IS MISLEADING TO suppose that women's health is dominated by hormones. On the contrary, it is women's general health, which is the result of lifestyle interacting with heredity, that determines hormonal health. Research has shown that eating for overall good health can improve menstrual and menopausal symptoms and can help prevent diseases such as breast cancer and osteoporosis. It also deeply affects the health of the next generation: the nutritional status of a woman at conception affects the risk of spina bifida, fetal brain development, and growth.

WOMEN'S HEALTH ❖ NEEDS ❖

Keeping active, with light exercise on a daily basis, is a crucial part of protecting your health. It allows you to eat more food, which improves nutrient intake, vital for general resistance to illness. Activity also guards against weight problems, diabetes, and high blood pressure. These all affect hormonal balance, which also influences bone strength. Establishing good eating and exercise habits early in life is the best way to prevent problems, but changes later in life are also worthwhile.

GENERAL ADVICE

• *Make nutrient-rich foods the basis of your diet, see the Basic Healthy Diet, pp. 12–13. Women need fewer calories than men, making it important for them to eat foods that supply a high level of vitamins and minerals per calorie.*
• *Eat plenty of iron-rich foods during your reproductive years. At this stage in life, women need almost twice as much iron a day as men to prevent iron deficiency or outright anemia, see p. 85.*
• *Many women are inactive. Make time to walk, especially up and down hills and stairs. Moderate weight-bearing exercise, such as housework, gardening, or carrying groceries, helps build and maintain strong bones.*
• *Avoid overstrenuous exercise and drastic dieting, both of which can disturb hormone metabolism, reducing bone strength and upsetting menstrual health.*
• *Do not smoke. Besides increasing the risk of many cancers, it doubles the risk of osteoporosis, reduces premenopausal protection against heart disease, and multiplies the risk of serious complications in pregnancy.*

PREMENSTRUAL SYNDROME

A few days before the commencement of menstruation, some women experience unpleasant symptoms such as fluid retention, see p. 84, irritability, fatigue, depression, constipation, and breast tenderness. This is due to imbalances of estrogen and progesterone, but the causes are not yet understood.

HELPFUL FOODS

• *Whole-wheat bread and cereals, soybeans, and crushed linseed* combine fiber with phytoestrogens, both thought to encourage the body to excrete surplus estrogen. Take ⅓ oz (9g) crushed linseed daily with 5fl oz (150ml) fluid. These foods can also relieve premenstrual constipation.
• *Wheat germ, potatoes, bananas, nuts, especially walnuts, red peppers, and cruciferous vegetables, especially raw*, are good sources of vitamin B6, which some women find helps their premenstrual symptoms. It may also be advisable to take supplements, which contain more vitamin B6 than you could obtain from food alone, but seek professional advice before taking them. About half of women who take supplements of 50mg or more a day have unwanted side effects.
• *Parsley, celery, artichokes, asparagus, and bitter salad greens* all stimulate urine production, which may help relieve fluid retention.

SUGAR-CRAVING

Many women feel hungrier, especially for sweet foods, in the 7–10 days before menstruating, and there is some evidence that the body uses up more calories at this time.
• To avoid eating too much sugar, eat small, frequent meals, focusing on foods that help keep blood sugar levels stable, see Blood Sugar Ratings, p. 91.

HELPFUL FOODS

• *Apples, pink grapefruit, plums, less ripe bananas, cherries, and dried apricots* are foods that taste sweet but cause blood sugar to rise and fall more gently than cookies, cakes, bread, or ripe bananas.

MENSTRUAL CRAMPS

These may be linked to anemia, see p. 85, and to poor circulation, see Circulation, pp. 82–5.

WEIGHT CONTROL

Obesity is a growing problem in industrialized countries and, paradoxically, so is the obsession with being thin. The best way of measuring whether your weight is healthy for your height is to work out your Body Mass Index, or BMI. The formula is:

$$\frac{\text{Weight in kilograms}}{\text{Height in meters squared}} = \text{BMI}$$

For example, someone who is 5ft 4in (1.63m) weighing 140lb (64kg) has a BMI of 24 (64 divided by 1.63^2).

If the answer to this sum is:
18 or less: you are underweight. Try not to let your weight fall further.
19–25: your weight comes within the healthy weight range.
26–30: you are overweight, which carries some extra health risk.
31 or more: you are obese and your health is definitely affected, with an increased risk of serious health problems.

ADVICE

• Whatever your weight, you should eat a nutritious diet, see the Basic Healthy Diet, pp. 12–13. If your BMI is 26 or more, you can lose weight healthily by eating more vegetables and fruit and less fat, see pp. 16–17. If your BMI is under 18, stress management, moderate exercise, and giving up smoking can help improve appetite and the body's utilization of food, and can help increase muscle size.

YEAST INFECTIONS

Weakness of the immune defenses, repeated use of antibiotics, and a lack of "friendly" bacteria in the body are mainly responsible for problems caused by the *Candida albicans* fungus, in the form of vaginal yeast infections. The fungus is present and harmless in most of us, unless the body's antifungal system allows it to grow too much.
• Limit use of antibiotics where possible. They kill "friendly" bacteria, which is thought to be a main cause of candida overgrowth.
• Some medicines, including oral contraceptives, may change the body's balance in a way that allows *Candida albicans* to increase.

HELPFUL FOODS

• *Yogurt with active* Lb. acidophilus *cultures* may help. In a trial, women with recurrent vaginal yeast infections who ate 8oz (225g) a day for a year had 3 times less infection. It may be worth trying live yogurt for thrush and other *Candida albicans* infections as well.
• *Garlic* has been shown to eliminate the *Candida albicans* fungus in animal and laboratory tests, but the effects on humans are not established.

BREAST CANCER RISK

There is increasing interest in the role of food in the risk of breast cancer. Although research is at a preliminary stage, it is currently thought that the risk may be reduced by a pattern of eating that is high in cereal fiber and in phytoestrogens, which are weak estrogenlike substances found in some plants. This advice is based on evidence that a woman is at greater risk of breast cancer when she has a high level of estrogen (or postmenopause, androgen) sex hormones circulating in her body. These levels may be reduced by eating larger amounts of cereal fiber, which appears to increase disposal of sex hormones, and eating more phytoestrogens, which are thought to supplant the body's own stronger estrogens, also reducing overall levels.

While premenopausal breast cancer is linked to being underweight, after menopause it is more common in overweight women. Weight gain in middle age, especially when it occurs around the waist, is associated with producing extra insulin after eating carbohydrates, and this may raise blood levels of estrogen and androgen sex hormones.
• Control your weight by eating less fat (except oily fish and linseed).
• Get regular exercise, which can help reduce insulin overproduction.

HELPFUL FOODS

• *Soybeans, tofu, soy flour and soy milk, linseed, fennel, legumes, whole wheat, barley, and green beans* are established phytoestrogenic foods. In a trial, women who ate 1½ oz (45g) a day of soy grits or soy flour for 12 weeks showed increased estrogen excretion.
• *Whole wheat and other unrefined grains* are the foods richest in insoluble fiber.

Women with a higher intake have been shown to have lower estrogen levels in the blood and a reduced risk of breast cancer.
• *Oats, legumes, pasta, whole-grain pumpernickel, vegetables, and fruits* are among the foods that produce a more gentle rise in blood sugar (compared with refined carbohydrates, sugar, and potatoes), which is less likely to provoke a high insulin response that can raise levels of sex hormones.

MENOPAUSAL CHANGES

In many women, the fluctuations in estrogen levels before menopause cause such symptoms as tiredness, hot flashes, broken sleep, and headaches. As estrogen stimulates bone mineralization, its decline during menopause increases the natural loss of bone density that occurs with age. In several recent studies, phytoestrogen-rich foods reduced menopausal hot flashes and reversed postmenopausal bone loss. Phytoestrogens are thought to work by mimicking estrogen.
• Eat a low-fat diet to guard against heart disease, see pp. 82–3, because women lose most of their protection from heart disease at menopause.
• Avoid becoming seriously overweight as it puts you at a much higher risk of stroke, diabetes, heart disease, arthritis, and breast cancer. If you have difficulty losing weight despite dieting, it may be due to the overproduction of insulin in reaction to eating refined carbohydrates. Choose carbohydrates that are least likely to have this effect, see Blood Sugar Ratings, p. 91.
• Do not take iron supplements unless you have a low hemoglobin level. After menopause, your iron needs almost halve and anemia is far less likely.
• Guard against osteoporosis, see p. 80.

HELPFUL FOODS

• *Soy grits and flour, linseed, crushed wheat grains, and unbleached white flour* are the most promising foods for reducing hot flashes that research has discovered so far. All of them substantially reduced hot flashes in trials on postmenopausal women when about 1½ oz (45g) a day was eaten for 12 weeks.
• *Fennel, cabbage, carrots, celery, cherries, nuts, parsley, sage, seeds, and spinach* also contain phytoestrogens, but their effects have not been tested.

SKIN

SKIN COMPLAINTS ARE SOME of the most common and difficult disorders to treat. Many problems are caused by adverse reactions to foods or chemicals, and the only treatment is to remove the cause. Most skin conditions, however, are signs of more general illness, and permanent relief requires tackling the underlying problem. Food can play a major part in skin health, helping prevent and relieve many ailments, but patience is needed.

❖ SKIN HEALTH ❖

The belief that eating mainly processed foods causes or worsens skin disorders has not been proved. However, eating mainly processed foods is unlikely to provide a good supply of nutrients, and they often have a high fat, sugar, and salt content that strains the body's health balance.

KEY NUTRIENTS

Zinc, vitamin A (both as retinol and as beta-carotene), vitamin E, and both essential fatty acids and their derivatives are especially good for skin health. They have all been convincingly linked to the prevention and treatment of many skin disorders. Rich sources are oysters, mussels, and other shellfish, liver, oily fish, lean meat, fruits and vegetables rich in beta-carotene, wheat germ, walnuts, sunflower seeds, and linseed.

ACNE

Acne is mainly linked to hormonal activity in the teens and early twenties.
• Avoid spreading the infection from one area of acne to another.
• Iodine can aggravate acne. Avoid fish, seafood, seaweed, and iodized salt for 2–3 weeks to see if acne improves.

HELPFUL FOODS

• *Foods rich in key nutrients for skin health, above,* provide the best support for healing.
• *Lean beef or lamb* is a good source of zinc. People prone to acne may need extra amounts. To aid zinc absorption, avoid bran, except in whole-wheat bread.

BOILS & CARBUNCLES

Boils and carbuncles, which are groups of boils, reflect a low resistance to infection. Recurrent boils may be a symptom of a more serious illness.

HELPFUL FOODS

• *Foods that support the body's defenses, see p. 89,* maximize resistance to infection.

ECZEMA

Extremely variable and often difficult to treat, eczema can be caused or worsened by an adverse reaction to irritants or food. There is often a family tendency to develop allergic reactions.
• Avoid possible irritants such as wool, nickel, and detergents.
• Identify possible problem foods such as milk, eggs, or wheat, see p. 79.
• The fatty acid, gamma-linolenic acid, from evening primrose oil and black currant seed oil may help relieve eczema. Try capsules containing these.

HELPFUL FOODS

• *Foods rich in key nutrients for skin health, above,* provide the best support for healing.
• *Wheat germ, linseed, finely ground black currants, sunflower seeds, watercress, and oily fish* contain fatty acids that may help relieve eczema.
• *Shellfish* is a good source of zinc. People prone to some forms of eczema may need extra amounts. Aid zinc absorption by avoiding bran except in whole-wheat bread.

PSORIASIS

This scaly skin condition is caused by skin cells reproducing too fast; it runs in families and is often linked to arthritis.
• Often, the most successful treatment for psoriasis is sunshine.
• Although psoriasis is notoriously difficult to treat, sufferers in some trials have improved on a low-protein, low-fat vegetarian diet of mainly brown rice and vegetables.
• It may help to keep intake of fat and omega-6 fatty acids low. These are high in most nuts, seeds, and vegetable oils.

HELPFUL FOODS

• *Oily fish and linseed* are the richest sources of omega-3 fatty acids, which are usually low in the skin of psoriasis sufferers. Daily therapy with the equivalent amount of fish oil obtained from a 5¼ oz (150g) serving of salmon or mackerel helped more than 50% of patients in one 8-week trial.
• *Artichokes, garlic, chili peppers, ginger, pineapple, and watercress* can aid poor digestion, which some natural practitioners believe underlies psoriasis.

WOUND-HEALING & BURNS

Help the healing of burns and wounds by drinking plenty of liquid.

HELPFUL FOODS

• *Liver, wheat germ, oysters and other shellfish, pineapple, green leafy vegetables, red peppers, walnuts, black currants, sunflower seeds, sweet potatoes, and pumpkin seeds* provide protein, folic acid, zinc, potassium, vitamin C, and essential fatty acids, which are needed for tissue replacement, and vitamin E, which has been confirmed to speed healing. Research on animals shows that it reduces inflammation and the formation of scar tissue. Pineapple enzymes can help reduce inflammation.

THE BODY'S DEFENSES

THE BODY HAS A SOPHISTICATED battery of defenses. In addition to the immune system, which fights harmful microorganisms, there are mechanisms to correct imbalances of fluid and to counter air pollutants, alcohol, and other substances that enter the body. The defense systems require many nutrients from food. Other special substances in some foods also seem to be able to help our defenses, whether against the common cold or the risk of many cancers.

❖ FIGHTING ❖ INFECTION

The immune system uses different types of white blood cells to destroy harmful microorganisms. It identifies them by their antigens, or chemical characteristics, and produces antibodies to attack them. In some cases, cancerous cells can also be detected and attacked. Once formed, antibodies protect us from getting certain diseases again. "Friendly" bacteria from some foods are thought to help the immune system fight some infections, such as yeast infections, see p. 87. Allergies are caused by the immune system over-reacting to certain foods, see p. 79.

GENERAL ADVICE

• *Maintain good hygiene habits. Reducing the number of micro-organisms entering the body lightens the workload of the immune system.*
• *Adopt a healthy lifestyle. Illness and some drugs, including alcohol and tobacco, reduce immune activity.*
• *Combat stress with yoga or meditation.*
• *Avoid heavy metals, such as lead (from old water pipes) and cadmium and mercury (from industrial pollution). These can depress immune action.*
• *Iron-deficiency anemia reduces resistance to infection, see p. 85.*

HELPFUL FOODS

• *Shellfish, chicken liver, oily fish, wheat germ, high-antioxidant vegetables and fruits such as carrots, sweet potatoes, and oranges, unrefined cereal grains, yogurt, sunflower seeds, and seaweed* are notable sources of nutrients especially linked with immune efficiency: the minerals zinc, calcium, copper, iodine, chromium, and magnesium; vitamins A, B6, folic acid, pantothenic acid, C, D, and E; and both essential fatty acids.
• *Yogurt with active cultures, garlic, cranberries, onion, chili peppers, honey, bilberries, and black currants* have all shown antibacterial action, and the first 3 are also antifungal. Live yogurt may work as a probiotic, encouraging beneficial bacteria in the intestine, see p. 23.
• *Garlic* has antiviral properties.
• *Tea* has been shown to combat the flu virus in laboratory tests.

❖ COPING WITH ❖ HARMFUL SUBSTANCES

Many threats to health come not from microorganisms but from substances such as tobacco smoke, too much salt, nitrates, alcohol, or excessive sunlight. The body needs substances from food to cope with these stresses. For example, people who eat too much salt need extra potassium to help dispose of it. Vitamin C is needed to counter the formation of potentially carcinogenic nitrate compounds, which can occur after we eat or drink nitrates in foods with fertilizer residues or preservatives, or in smoked food.

GENERAL ADVICE

• *Try to reduce contact with substances that increase the load on the body's defenses, such as tobacco smoke, car fumes, and excess alcohol.*

HELPFUL FOODS

• *Green leafy vegetables, carrots, red peppers, sweet potatoes, citrus fruits, whole-grain cereals, sunflower seeds, oysters, and other shellfish* are rich sources of the antioxidants beta-carotene, vitamins E and C, and the minerals selenium and zinc (see also pp. 144–9 for other good food sources). A plentiful supply of antioxidants from food is important to help the body counter potentially harmful free radicals that result from oxidation, see Antioxidants, p. 21. In excess, free radicals are a danger associated with heart disease and some forms of cancer. Air pollutants, smoke, and excessive sunlight can multiply the free radicals that the body must deal with. People who eat high levels of vegetables and fruits have lower levels of heart disease, stroke, cataracts, and some forms of cancer.
• *Onions, garlic, and cruciferous vegetables such as cabbage* contain sulfur compounds that are thought to counter some carcinogens. In diet surveys, people who eat more of these foods show lower rates of some cancers.
• *Onions, tea (green or black), and red wine* are the richest common sources of quercetin, a flavonoid with an antioxidant action recently linked to a lower risk of heart disease and stroke.
• *Fruits and vegetables* contain many other flavonoids, see p. 22. Most have not yet been researched, but some that have, such as the anthocyanin flavonoids found in bilberries, have shown an antioxidant action. The presence of flavonoids and other special substances may partly explain why antioxidants taken as supplements do not show the same protective effects as eating vegetables and fruits.

DIABETIC HEALTH

 DIABETES OCCURS WHEN THE body has lost the ability to keep its blood sugar level within the range needed for good health. It is a growing risk for middle-aged people in developed countries due to lack of activity and serious obesity. Even with treatment, diabetics must take diet and exercise seriously to avoid poor blood sugar control damaging their circulation and risking sight damage, heart disease, foot gangrene, and kidney failure. The lifestyle that is beneficial for diabetics can also prevent many people from developing diabetes in middle age and can improve general health.

❖ DIABETES ❖

The body breaks down starch and sugar into basic sugars for digestion. Normally, when this sugar is absorbed into the bloodstream, the pancreas produces the right amount of the hormone insulin to allow the sugar to leave the bloodstream to be used as energy or stored. In diabetes, the body may stop producing insulin, produce too little, or produce plenty but become insulin-resistant and unable to use it. Absence of usable insulin means the body cannot use most of the carbohydrate eaten. In addition to affecting energy, this disrupts many body systems, especially circulation.

So far, ways of preventing diabetes in children or young adults are unknown; more treatments are now being researched. Although diabetes tends to run in families, by middle age, being seriously overweight multiplies your risk of the disorder, and new cases are twice as common among inactive people.

.... *Caution* ....
The type of diabetes most common in young people is so life-threatening that it is usually diagnosed quickly, but diabetes that appears in middle age can be missed. Seek urgent professional advice for symptoms such as tiredness, dizziness, excessive thirst, recurrent pins and needles, blurred vision, or frequent urination.

GENERAL ADVICE

• *Avoid becoming seriously overweight, see Weight Control, p. 87, especially if you know of diabetes in your family, or have had a baby weighing 10lb (4.5kg) or more: a marker of higher future risk. Being overweight, especially around the waist, leads to insulin resistance.*
• *Regular light exercise improves the body's ability to use its insulin.*
• *Avoid eating concentrated sugar or low-fiber carbohydrates without "padding" them with soluble fiber or resistant starch, both of which slow the rise in blood sugar. The soluble fiber in oat bran muffins, for example, helps to counteract the effect of their sugar content.*

CONTROLLING BLOOD SUGAR LEVELS

Most young diabetics require prescribed insulin throughout their lives, but in middle age, being overweight can trigger insulin-resistant diabetes in some people who produce plenty of insulin. With exercise and weight loss under medical supervision, they can use more of their own insulin and balance their blood sugar by diet alone. All diabetics have to balance the amount of carbohydrates they eat with the amount of energy they use in activity and their available insulin, natural or prescribed. Diabetics are advised to eat much the same pattern of food as other people: low in fat, high in fiber, with unrefined carbohydrates, vegetables, and fruits (see the Basic

Healthy Diet, pp. 12–13), emphasizing foods that help blood sugar control.
• Cut your intake of sugar to 1oz (25g) maximum. Spread your allowance over the day, and eat it with foods high in soluble fiber. Fructose sugar does not require insulin for absorption and, used in small amounts, is the best choice for table sugar.
• Favor foods that produce smaller rises in blood sugar, see p. 91.
• Where possible, avoid foods that raise blood sugar more sharply. These include fine-textured wheat bread, even when whole wheat, cornflakes, carrots, pumpkin, ripe bananas, and potatoes.
• Replace 3 meals a day with 6 mini-meals to help to steady blood sugar.

HELPFUL FOODS

• *Rolled oats, oat bran, and oatmeal (not instant oat cereal), onions, artichokes, and legumes* are foods that have shown an ability to reduce blood sugar rises.
• *Shellfish, lean meat, whole-grain cereals, legumes, pumpkin seeds, and nuts* combine chromium and zinc, 2 minerals often low in diabetics. Chromium is central to normal functioning of the insulin mechanism, and zinc is important for resistance to infection, which is abnormally low in many diabetics.
• *Wheat germ, less ripe bananas, turkey, fish, nuts, especially walnuts, red peppers, and cruciferous vegetables* are good sources of vitamin B_6, needed for blood sugar control. Many diabetics have low levels of this nutrient.

CIRCULATION DISORDERS

Poor circulation affects many diabetics. Minimizing damage depends on the control of blood sugar levels. Circulation damage increases the risk of heart disease and can be a cause of neuropathy (damage to the nerves of the peripheries), which can lead to sight loss, gangrene, and impotence.

• Do not smoke: it damages circulation.
• Avoid constriction around the extremities.
• Supplements from black currant seeds or evening primrose containing gamma-linolenic acid (GLA) can help diabetic neuropathy. Try 360mg GLA a day.

HELPFUL FOODS

• *Wheat germ, sunflower seeds, canola oil, almonds, and sweet potatoes* contain high levels of vitamin E. Substantial research has shown that this improves diabetic circulation and can help diabetic neuropathy. Although research used supplements of 400mg a day, which is far more than you could obtain from food, eating plenty of foods rich in vitamin E has proved valuable in reducing the risk of cataracts, to which diabetics are especially prone.
• *Bilberries* contain anthocyanin flavonoids, which in trials have helped diabetic retinopathy and peripheral circulation by improving capillary wall resistance to blood leakage.
• *Blueberries, black currants, red or black cherries, black raspberries, and cranberries* also contain anthocyanins, but their effects have not been tested. Black currants are rich in vitamin C, which is also needed for cell wall strength

❖ HEALTHY EATING PLAN ❖

These are examples of meals including foods that can benefit diabetics and help regulate blood sugar. This style of eating may also benefit nondiabetics by helping avoid high blood insulin levels, which are linked to being overweight in middle age and a higher risk of heart disease and breast cancer.

Breakfasts
• Oatmeal with added oat bran and wheat germ
Apple or grapefruit

• Low-fat yogurt with sunflower seeds and dried apricot purée

• Baked beans on whole-grain toast with grilled tomatoes
Blueberries

• Real Muesli, p. 131
Lean bacon and poached egg
Orange or grapefruit

Snacks
• Oat Bran Muffins, p. 137; apples; sunflower seeds; dried apricots; almonds; celery stalks

Light Meals
• Lentil soup
Waldorf Salad, p. 110

• Rye pumpernickel
Green bean and corn salad
Swiss Onion Soup, p. 102

• Celery and walnut sandwich made with mixed grain bread

• Suimono Soup, p. 101
Artichoke Heart Salad, p. 109

• Tabbouleh, p. 113, with salsa
Chicken with Slaw Salad, p. 112

Main Meals
• Artichokes with vinaigrette made with sunflower oil
Salmon Kedgeree, p. 116, served with Pineapple Salsa, p. 138, and green beans
Kissel, p. 133, made with blueberries

• Lima Beans with Sage & Garlic, p. 125
Forty-Clove Garlic Chicken, p. 117, served with barley and almonds; green salad
Fresh plums or cherries

• Nut & Cherry Pilaf, p. 123, made with bulgur wheat, served with Sunflower Green Salad, p. 112
Baked apples stuffed with dried pears

• Onions à la Grecque, p. 107
Greek Fish Stew, p. 115, served with red cabbage
Summer Pudding, p. 129, made with plums and berries

• Warm Walnut Dip with Grilled Vegetables, p. 105
Falafel, p. 123, and Low-Fat Hummus, p. 140, with cucumber salad
Apricot Almond Fool, p. 130

• Shiro Ae Salad, p. 111
Broccoli Stir-Fry, p. 121, made with almonds
Cranberry & Apricot Compote, p. 132

❖ BLOOD SUGAR RATINGS ❖

This table compares how much blood sugar rises in groups of diabetics and nondiabetics after eating various carbohydrate foods. Figures are measured against eating the equivalent amount of glucose, which is counted as 100%. The lower the number, the less the food raises blood sugar. Foods that are low in sugar, high in soluble fiber or resistant starch, and composed of larger particles generally score best.

• *Glucose*	100%
• *Grains*	
Pasta, whole-wheat or white	42–50
Rice, brown or white	47–55
Oat muesli (package)	60
Cooked Oatmeal	49
Bread, whole-wheat or white	70–78
Bread, mixed grain or pumpernickel	45
Cornflakes	78
• *Sugars*	
Fructose	20
Sucrose	65

• *Legumes*	
Soybeans, lentils, chickpeas, baked beans	20–40
• *Fruit*	
Cherries, grapefruit, dried apricots	32 or less
Oranges, apples, pears	36–43
Bananas, depending on ripeness	30–70
• *Vegetables*	
All very low except peas, sweet potatoes, corn	48–55
Potatoes, carrots	56–85

KIDNEYS & URINARY SYSTEM

 THE HEALTH OF THE KIDNEYS and urinary tract is directly affected by what we eat and drink. The kidneys filter some 47 gallons of body fluids a day, and any faltering in their function rapidly affects the body's fluid balance, which is central to health. The kidneys also affect the production of hormones and red blood cells. Men can help general urinary health by eating to discourage enlargement of the prostate, which causes some urinary obstruction in most older men.

❖ KIDNEYS ❖

The kidneys maintain the body's delicate balance of fluid and acid and alkaline constituents by disposing of surplus water, sodium, potassium, and other elements. They also help determine bone strength, activate vitamin D, and make a hormone needed for red blood cell production. Poor kidney function can lead to anemia, weaker bones, water retention, high blood pressure, a greater risk of general infection, and kidney stones.

GENERAL ADVICE

• *Drink about 6 glasses (1½ liters) of fluid a day to help the kidneys dilute the substances they must excrete.*
• *Avoid an excessive intake of salt, protein, and sugar, each of which puts an extra load on the kidneys.*

HELPFUL FOODS

• *Dried apricots, green leafy vegetables, potatoes, and bananas* are rich in potassium, an ample supply of which helps the kidneys excrete the excessive amount of sodium found in a typical Western-style diet.
• *Asparagus, celery, parsley, artichokes, and black currants* have gentle diuretic properties, which help the kidneys dispose of body wastes by encouraging urine production.

--------------- *Caution* ---------------
Gout sufferers should not eat asparagus.

KIDNEY STONES

A growing number of people develop kidney stones, which often recur. There is so much calcium oxalate compound or uric acid in their urine that it forms crystals. When these pass down the urinary tract they cause pain, vomiting, and scarring. Known causal factors are a Western-style diet and too little urine to dilute stone ingredients. This may occur after dehydration, or infections that affect kidney efficiency.
• Avoid softened drinking water: people living in soft-water areas have a higher kidney stone risk.
• Stones are much more common in those who eat meat than in vegetarians.
• The stones of most sufferers contain calcium oxalate. High levels of this in the urine can be caused by poor digestion. Even though most oxalate is made in the body, if you have passed a stone containing this mineral, limit oxalate derived from food by avoiding spinach, rhubarb, and large amounts of strong black tea or cranberries.
• Drinking 2–2½ quarts (2–2½ liters) of fluid a day is the most effective way to prevent more stones from forming.

HELPFUL FOODS

• *Whole-grain cereals, wheat germ, nuts, and seeds* are rich in magnesium and fiber, which makes it easier for the body to excrete excess calcium and oxalate.
• *Wheat germ, bananas, potatoes, walnuts, red peppers, and cruciferous vegetables* are high in vitamin B6, which helps the body dispose of oxalate harmlessly.
• *Cranberries,* in moderate amounts (of juice or berries), may help prevent calcium stones recurring by lowering calcium levels in urine.

❖ URINARY TRACT ❖

Urine leaving the kidneys trickles down two ureter passages, to be stored in the bladder until it is urinated through the urethra passage. A free flow of urine is important for both sexes, helping prevent infection by washing out bacteria and minerals that can form bladder stones.

GENERAL ADVICE

• *Do not resist the need to urinate.*

URINARY TRACT INFECTIONS

Infections of the urinary passages and bladder are usually caused by bacteria from the anus being transferred to the urethra, a short distance in women. Preventing transfer is a key protective measure. Bladder infection, or cystitis, not only is painful, but, if recurrent, can lead to kidney infection.
• Try to drink at least 3 quarts (3 liters) of water a day during infection.

HELPFUL FOODS

• *Foods that support the body's defenses, p. 89,* help reduce the risk of infection.
• *Cranberries and blueberries* help prevent bacteria from adhering to the walls of the urethra and bladder. 10fl oz (300ml) of cranberry juice or 3oz (85g) fresh cranberries a day are effective ways to reduce the risk of infection. 14–18fl oz (340–500ml) of juice or 2 large helpings of berries a day can relieve symptoms.
• *Garlic* has a general antibacterial effect that can help prevent infection.

❖ ENLARGED PROSTATE ❖

Most men develop some enlargement of the prostate gland between the ages of 40 and 60. The resulting pressure on the urethra can cause frequent and sometimes painful urination, slow passing of urine, and difficulty in emptying the bladder completely. This increases the risk of bladder infection and stones.

GENERAL ADVICE

• *Watch your weight. A large abdomen puts pressure on the bladder.*

HELPFUL FOODS

• *Oysters, whelks, and other shellfish, lean meat, pine nuts, sesame seeds, tahini, and pecans* are rich in zinc, ample amounts of which are required for normal prostate function.
• *Wheat germ, oily fish, and linseed* provide omega-3 fatty acids and omega-6 fatty acids, which can both have an anti-inflammatory action.
• *Pumpkin seeds* are traditionally used to counter prostate enlargement. They combine zinc with anti-inflammatory fatty acids and a phytosterol that is thought to reduce a hormone reaction that causes prostate swelling. Eat 1–1¾oz (25–50g) a day, chewing well, or grind in a blender.
• *Parsley* is another traditional prostate remedy, probably because it has a diuretic effect. It is useful both fresh and dried. Try about 1oz (25g) fresh leaves a day.

EMOTIONAL HEALTH

THE FOODS WE EAT can affect our emotional state in several ways, and vice versa. We all know this, at least subconsciously, from our observations of how hunger makes people bad-tempered, or how people use food to cheer themselves up. Popular images of "comfort food" are not all in the mind: connections between food and mood are increasingly backed by research, suggesting that many of us subconsciously choose certain foods for their effects on our mood and emotions.

❖ DIET & EMOTIONS ❖

The most direct way that food influences mood is via its effect on blood sugar. Many people's mood deteriorates as their blood sugar level falls. The type of food eaten matters too. There is increasing evidence that eating foods high in carbohydrates but low in protein, such as candies and chocolate, can lift mood and increase calmness and drowsiness. It is thought that, as long as there is not much protein present, the insulin released by eating carbohydrates triggers an increase in the level of the calming neurotransmitter, serotonin, in the brain. Carbohydrate foods that contain tryptophan, the precursor of serotonin, are most likely to have this effect, and a few foods contain serotonin itself. Mood and emotions may also be affected by a shortage of certain nutrients; for example, iron deficiency can result in depression.

Individual sensitivity to certain foods can cause behavioral changes and mood changes, such as hyperactivity.

GENERAL ADVICE

• *You may improve your emotional balance by observing how your mood affects what you eat and vice versa.*
• *Restrict "comfort" eating to carbohydrates that are unrefined and low in fat. Otherwise, you risk becoming overweight, which affects heart health.*
• *If your mood slumps after eating, steady your blood sugar level by spreading food over 5–6 light meals a day rather than 2–3 heavy ones.*

MOODINESS, RESTLESSNESS, NERVOUSNESS & SLEEP PROBLEMS

You can help relieve these symptoms, usually thought to be "all in the mind," by eating to obtain a high intake of iron, vitamins B1, B2, niacin, vitamin B6, folic acid, vitamin C, zinc, and magnesium, and by stabilizing your blood sugar level.
• *Liver, wheat germ, green leafy vegetables, peas, shellfish, game, oily fish, nuts, and seeds* are rich in nutrients, *above*, related to mood and emotional state. Try to eat more of them when under stress, after illness, or taking medication, all of which can affect digestion, reducing the absorption of some nutrients.
• *Bananas* contain some serotonin, and are a more nourishing way of improving mood than confectionery or sugary pastries. Eating 1–2 bananas without other food has been shown to increase serotonin in the body.
• *Oats* are used by herbalists as a "nerve nourisher," but it is not known how it works.
• *Lettuce, celery, and asparagus* have traditionally been eaten to produce a sedative effect. A sedative substance has been found in celery, and a soporific one in lettuce.
• *Unrefined carbohydrates, especially oats and barley, legumes, fruits, and vegetables*, are high in soluble fiber and help stabilize blood sugar levels, see Diabetes, pp. 90–1.

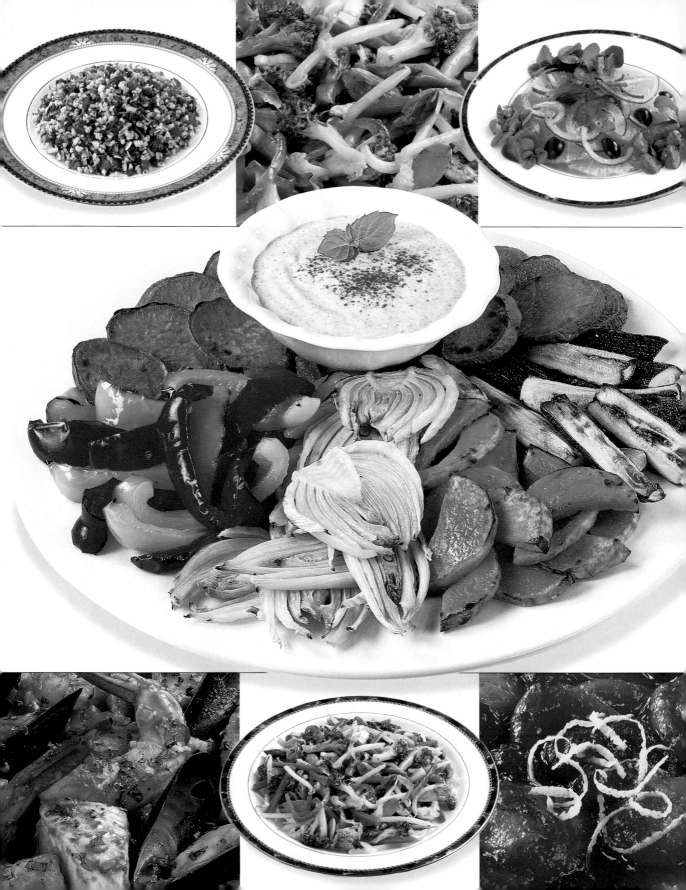

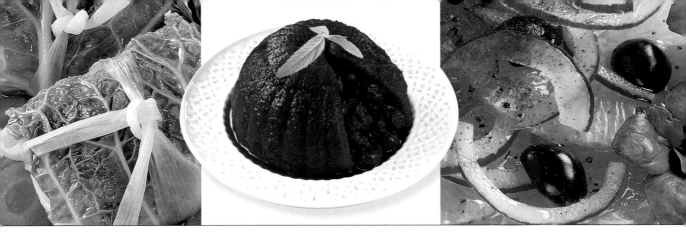

RECIPES

The recipes in this section show how the 50 key foods

can be enjoyed in ethnic, modern, and classic dishes.

All are designed to fit into a well-balanced eating style,

to retain health value in preparation, and to taste good.

All the dishes serve 4, unless otherwise indicated.
Nutritional data are approximate due to the natural variation
in the nutrient levels of food, see p. 160.

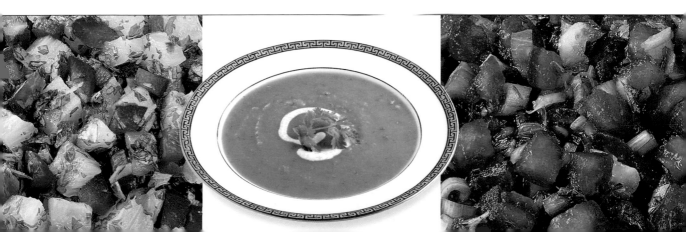

THE HEALTHY KITCHEN

MANY OF THE HEALTH benefits of food depend on how it is stored and prepared. Certain items of kitchen equipment and methods of cooking also assist healthier eating. An important first step toward enjoying the health benefits of food is to select good ingredients. When possible, choose organically grown ingredients and lower-fat meat and dairy products, see p. 13. Since most of the salt we eat comes from ready-made foods, you can eat less salt by cooking with fresh foods and using flavorings such as herbs, spices, citrus zest and juice, garlic, and nuts.

❖ PREPARATION ❖

RETAINING MORE NUTRIENTS
Chop vegetables, fruits, herbs, nuts, and seeds as close to cooking or serving time as possible to avoid exposing the cut surfaces of food to the destructive effects of air, light, and heat, which reduce nutrients in food, mainly by oxidation, see p. 21. Chopping also releases an enzyme that kills vitamin C. Coat cut surfaces with citrus juice, which is antioxidant, or use a tight cover. Do not soak prepared produce; water-soluble nutrients will leach away.

Mezzaluna
A crescent-shaped rocking knife is very useful for chopping large amounts of fresh herbs, such as parsley, easily.

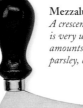

Swivel-bladed peeler
A sharp peeler removes a very thin layer of peel and retains the highly nutritious layer under the skin.

Stiff brush
Before using fruit peel, scrub fruits in hot, soapy water to help remove wax and sprays, then rinse. Produce, too, can simply be scrubbed instead of peeled.

Food processor
By making it easier to chop fresh ingredients just before cooking, a food processor reduces the loss of nutrients by oxidation.

STORAGE

Polyunsaturated fats, especially if low in antioxidant vitamin E, are prone to oxidation and turn rancid more quickly when exposed to air, heat, and light. Improve the oxidation resistance of vulnerable oils, such as walnut, by breaking a capsule of vitamin E into the bottle when it is first opened.

Avoid food packaged in plastic or stored in contact with plastic, especially fatty foods, such as cheese, processed meats or oils, and alcoholic drinks: this eliminates the possible transfer of harmful chemicals from the plastic.

Airtight dark glass and stainless steel containers
To avoid turning polyunsaturate-rich nuts, seeds, wheat germ, and vegetable oils into potential health hazards, keep them in airtight containers in a cool, dark place and use them as quickly as possible.

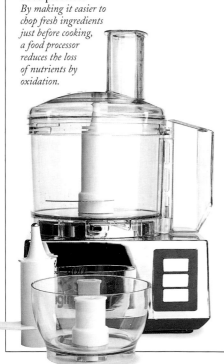

❖ COOKING EQUIPMENT ❖

HEALTHIER COOKWARE

Stainless-steel, cast-iron, or glass cookware is best for health. The suggested link between aluminum cookware and Alzheimer's disease has not been proved, but it is a legitimate concern. A pan with a heavy base spreads heat evenly, allowing you to cook with less fat without food burning. Cast-iron pans conduct heat very well. Stainless steel conducts heat poorly, so choose pans lined with an enclosed layer of copper or aluminum in the base, which improves heat conduction.

Briefly cooking vegetables retains more vitamins and minerals

Tight-fitting lid
A tight lid conserves nutrients by holding in steam and heat. This shortens cooking time and, when cooking vegetables, reduces the amount of water needed.

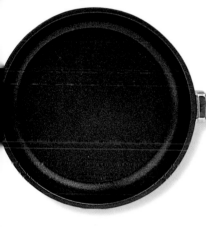

Pan with a nonstick finish
A nonstick finish on the pan aids low-fat cooking, but if the finish is scratched or shows signs of peeling, discard the pan.

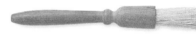

Natural bristle brush
A brush dipped in oil coats skillets or baking pans with a minimum amount of fat. Plastic bristle brushes will melt when in contact with a hot pan.

COOKING TIPS

All cooking of fruits and vegetables causes some loss of nutrients, but the amount varies according to the length of time food is heated and how long it is in contact with water.

MINIMIZE HEATING TIME
• Boil water before adding fruits or vegetables (even potatoes) to the pan.
• Cover the pan or steamer tightly to prevent steam from escaping during cooking.
• Cook food for the shortest possible time (a timer is essential).
• Avoid keeping hot food waiting.

LIMIT THE LOSS OF NUTRIENTS
• Steaming and boiling with a little water have equally good results; steaming prevents nutrients from draining away into the cooking water, whereas boiling heats food more quickly to the cooking temperature at which a vitamin C–destroying enzyme is killed.
• When boiling, use only a 1 inch (2–3cm) depth of water.
• Retrieve lost nutrients by using cooking water as stock.
• Do not salt cooking water – it draws water from food, which carries away nutrients as well.
• Never add baking soda when cooking vegetables to keep them green: it destroys vitamin C.

• Pressure cookers and microwave ovens can help retain nutrients because they shorten cooking (if carefully timed) and reduce the need to add water.

WHICH OIL?
Cold-pressed, unrefined oils retain more nutritional value and flavor.

For high-temperature cooking

Olive, canola, and sesame oils

For low-temperature cooking

Sunflower, hazelnut, and canola oils

For cold dishes

Sunflower, hazelnut, wheat germ, walnut, and olive oils

SOUPS

SOUPS ARE AN ENJOYABLE, valuable, and delicious way to eat more nutritionally rich foods and can be particularly beneficial for people with small appetites for vegetables, who would otherwise never eat such a generous helping of these vital foods. Today's soups have even more food value, thanks to the arrival of blenders. Now velvet-smooth vegetable soups need only the briefest cooking, conserving their heat-sensitive vitamins and appetizing bright colors. Not only do the vegetables keep their flavor better but the soup gets all the smoothness it needs from blending, so the old reliance on butter and cream is obsolete, and less salt is needed. Blenders make soup-making a less labor-intensive undertaking. Ingredients no longer need to be chopped so fine or by hand, so busy cooks can make soups more often. Warming, nourishing, filling, and easily kept low in calories, these soups are also useful for people who want to lose weight.

RED FRUIT SOUP
This traditional Northern
European soup contains
very little fat.

*The soup's color will
range from bright pink
to blue–black, depending
on the berries you choose*

❖ RED FRUIT SOUP ❖

INGREDIENTS

1lb 2oz (500g) mixed berries, such as bilberries, blueberries, cherries, black currants, and cranberries, fresh, frozen, or canned in unsweetened juice, drained weight

2¼ cups (500ml) water or juice from canned fruit

zest of 1 lemon

1 cinnamon stick

2 cloves

honey, to taste

4 tsp crème fraîche or sour cream, to garnish

This chilled soup is a refreshing first course to serve before a substantial main course. Mixing tart and sweet berries reduces the need for sweetening.

1 Remove any stems or seeds from the fresh fruit and rinse gently under running water. Let drain. Frozen berries can be used straight from the freezer.
2 In a large pan, heat the water or juice with the zest, cinnamon, and cloves and simmer for about 10 minutes. Discard the spices, retain the zest, and add the fruit.
3 Cook the fruit for 3–10 minutes, or until just soft. Purée the soup in a blender or food processor until smooth. Chill for 2 hours before serving.
4 After 1 hour, add the honey to taste. The soup should have a tart flavor. Garnish each serving with a swirl of crème fraîche or sour cream.

NUTRITIONAL INFORMATION

Amount per serving

Calories (kcal)	69
Total fat (g)	1
% of calories	14
Sat. fat (g)	1
% of calories	8
Cholesterol (mg)	3
Total carb. (g)	14
Starch (g)	0
Fiber (g)	3
Protein (g)	1
Sodium (mg)	5

Rich source of vitamin C

HEALTH LINKS

Gastroenteritis, p. 79
Circulation, pp. 82–5
Urinary tract infections, p. 92

❖ HOT & SOUR SOUP ❖

INGREDIENTS

½ cup (25g) dried Chinese mushrooms

¼ tsp sea salt

¼ tsp brown sugar

1 tsp light soy sauce

1 tsp dry sherry

4 tsp potato starch

1 tbsp water

1 tsp sesame oil

¼ lb (100g) lean pork strips

⅓ lb (180g) firm tofu

5 cups (1.2 liters) chicken stock

3 tbsp light soy sauce

2 eggs, beaten

3 tbsp sweet rice vinegar

2 tbsp chopped fresh cilantro

freshly ground black pepper

1 tsp sesame oil

2 scallions, trimmed and cut into ½ inch (1cm) slices

1–2 tsp chili oil

Surprisingly uncomplicated to make, this warming but not too fiery Chinese broth is a tasty way to eat tofu. A large bowlful makes a light meal.

1 Place the dried mushrooms in a heatproof bowl and cover with boiling water. Let stand for 30 minutes.
2 Make a marinade by mixing the salt, sugar, soy sauce, sherry, starch, water, and oil in a glass bowl.
3 Add the pork strips to the marinade and let stand for 20 minutes.
4 Drain and dice the tofu. Any liquid from the drained tofu can go into the soup. Drain and slice the mushrooms into very thin strips.
5 In a large saucepan, bring the stock to a boil. Add the soy sauce, mushrooms, and the marinade with the pork strips. Cook for a few minutes, then reduce the heat.
6 Add the tofu and gently return the mixture to a boil to avoid breaking up the cubes of tofu.
7 Gradually pour in the eggs over the back of a fork, gently stirring the soup with the fork at the same time to separate the egg strands. Turn off the heat and allow the eggs to set for a minute.
8 Stir in the vinegar, cilantro, pepper, and sesame oil. Taste and add a little more soy sauce or vinegar if you prefer.
9 Sprinkle a few scallions and some chili oil in each bowl. Pour the hot soup over and serve.

NUTRITIONAL INFORMATION

Amount per serving

Calories (kcal)	182
Total fat (g)	11
% of calories	54
Sat. fat (g)	2
% of calories	11
Cholesterol (mg)	114
Total carb. (g)	7
Starch (g)	1
Fiber (g)	trace
Protein (g)	14
Sodium (mg)	875

Rich source of calcium, phosphorus

HEALTH LINKS

Respiratory infections, p. 76
Digestion, pp. 78–9
Circulation, pp. 82–5
Menopause, p. 87

❖ CARROT & CILANTRO SOUP ❖

INGREDIENTS

2¼ lb (1kg) carrots
1 tbsp olive oil or 1 tbsp butter, or a mixture
5 cups (1.2 liters) water or meat or vegetable stock
4 tsp chopped fresh cilantro
freshly ground black pepper
sea salt
4 tsp sour cream, to garnish

This colorful smooth-textured soup can provide the vegetable part of a meal and is practical for picnics or as a snack.

1 Peel the carrots unless they are organic, in which case they can be scraped or scrubbed instead. Cut into chunks.
2 In a large saucepan, heat the oil or butter, add the carrots, and cook gently for a few minutes.
3 Add the water or stock, bring to a boil, cover, reduce the heat, and simmer for 15 minutes.
4 Using a blender or food processor, purée the carrots and cooking liquid with the cilantro, reserving a few leaves for the garnish. Season to taste. Garnish each serving with a swirl of sour cream.

NUTRITIONAL INFORMATION

Amount per serving

Calories (kcal)	13
Total fat (g)	(
% of calories	38
Sat. fat (g)	
% of calories	1(
Cholesterol (mg)	
Total carb. (g)	2(
Starch (g)	
Fiber (g)	(
Protein (g)	2
Sodium (mg)	66

Rich source of carotenes, potassium

HEALTH LINKS

Heart health, pp. 82–5
The body's defenses, p. 89

VARIATIONS

◆ *Use the same method to make fennel or beet soup.*
◆ *Replace the cilantro with other fresh herbs, such as dill, chives, lemon thyme, or fennel.*

❖ SUIMONO SOUP ❖

INGREDIENTS

4½ cups (1 liter) water
½ oz (15g) kombu seaweed
½ oz (15g) shaved dried bonito fillet (katsuobushi)
2 tsp light soy sauce
9oz (250g) firm tofu
2 scallions, finely chopped
lemon zest

VARIATIONS

◆ Replace the tofu with cooked, thinly sliced chicken, shrimp, or other shellfish. Simmer the soup for a few extra minutes to cook.
◆ Replace the scallions with sprigs of watercress, shredded nori, thin slices of leek, or a few green peas.

This clear, almost fat-free Japanese broth balances a substantial main course or a rich dessert.

1 Bring the water to a boil. Add the seaweed, reduce the heat, and simmer for 4 minutes, stirring continuously.
2 Using a slotted spoon, remove the seaweed and add the bonito shavings. Return to a boil, then remove the pan from the heat. When the bonito shavings settle to the bottom of the pan, strain the broth, or *dashi*, and discard the bonito shavings.
3 Return the broth to a boil and add the soy sauce to taste.
4 Drain and cut the tofu into 8 cubes. Add to the broth and heat gently, to avoid breaking up the cubes of tofu, until very hot.
5 Add a sprinkling of scallions, a strip of lemon zest, and 2 cubes of tofu to each soup bowl. Pour the hot broth over and serve immediately.

NUTRITIONAL INFORMATION

Amount per serving	
Calories (kcal)	49
Total fat (g)	3
% of calories	49
Sat. fat (g)	1
% of calories	6
Cholesterol (mg)	0
Total carb. (g)	1
Starch (g)	trace
Fiber (g)	2
Protein (g)	6
Sodium (mg)	273
Rich source of calcium, iodine	

HEALTH LINK

Menopause, p. 87

❖ SPICED CHICKEN COCONUT SOUP ❖

INGREDIENTS

4½ cups (1 liter) water
1 chicken breast, including the skin and bones
1 onion, chopped
4 kaffir lime leaves
3 stems lemongrass, lightly crushed
1½ inch (3cm) piece fresh ginger or 4 inch (10cm) piece fresh galangal, thinly sliced
1 small red chili pepper, seeded and finely sliced
¼ lb (100g) oyster or shiitake mushrooms, thinly sliced
2 water chestnuts, thinly sliced, optional
1 tbsp Thai fish sauce
juice of 1 lime and ½ lemon
scant 1 cup (200ml) coconut milk
freshly ground black pepper
sea salt
2 tbsp chopped fresh cilantro

Chili pepper, onion, and ginger are combined to make this substantial Thai-style soup, which stimulates the circulation and helps the digestion.

1 In a large saucepan, heat the water with the chicken, onion, lime leaves, lemongrass, ginger, and chili pepper. Bring to a boil, cover tightly, reduce the heat, and simmer for 20 minutes, until the chicken is tender.
2 Lift out the chicken breast, remove the skin and bones, and slice the meat. Return the skin and bones to the broth and simmer for another 15 minutes.
3 Strain the broth. Discard the spices, except for a few slices of chili pepper, which add color to the soup. Return the broth to the pan. Add the chicken meat, mushrooms, and water chestnuts, if using.
4 Simmer for 3 minutes, then add the fish sauce, lime and lemon juice, and coconut milk. Remove from the heat and season to taste.
5 Add some chopped cilantro to each soup bowl. Reheat the soup but do not boil. Pour over and serve.

NUTRITIONAL INFORMATION

Amount per serving	
Calories (kcal)	83
Total fat (g)	6
% of calories	60
Sat. fat (g)	4
% of calories	44
Cholesterol (mg)	16
Total carb. (g)	1
Starch (g)	trace
Fiber (g)	trace
Protein (g)	7
Sodium (mg)	202

HEALTH LINKS

Respiratory infections, p. 76
Digestion, pp. 78–9
Circulation, pp. 82–5

VARIATION

◆ Add ½ lb (200g) cubed tofu with the chicken in step 3.

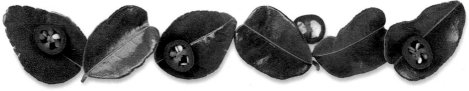

❖ GREEN SHCHI SOUP ❖

INGREDIENTS

2 eggs, optional

5 cups (1.2 liters) vegetable stock

1 celery stalk, finely sliced

1 bay leaf

5 peppercorns, any color

1 onion, finely chopped

½ lb (200g) potatoes, diced

2 tbsp kasha or rice, optional

1lb 2oz (500g) spinach or sorrel or young nettle leaves, or a mixture

2 tbsp chopped fresh dill, optional

squeeze of lemon juice

sea salt

4 tsp sour cream, to garnish

This meatless version of a traditional Russian soup is adaptable to whatever leafy greens are in season and is a good way to eat these protective foods.

1 Hard-cook the eggs, if using, drain, and let stand in cold water.

2 In a large saucepan, heat the stock with the celery, bay leaf, peppercorns, onion, potato, and kasha or rice, if using. When the mixture comes to a boil, reduce the heat and simmer, covered, for 15 minutes.

3 Meanwhile, wash the spinach or other leafy greens thoroughly and chop. Remove the bay leaf and peppercorns from the pan, add the spinach or other leafy greens, and return the mixture to a boil.

4 Cook for 2 minutes, then remove from the heat. Let stand, covered, for 5 minutes.

5 In a blender or food processor, purée all or part of the spinach mixture, according to preference. Add the dill, if using, the lemon juice, and salt to taste.

6 Garnish each serving with a dollop of sour cream, topped with half a hard-boiled egg, if using, and serve.

NUTRITIONAL INFORMATION

Amount per serving

Calories (kcal)	91
Total fat (g)	2
% of calories	22
Sat. fat (g)	1
% of calories	7
Cholesterol (mg)	3
Total carb. (g)	13
Starch (g)	8
Fiber (g)	4
Protein (g)	5
Sodium (mg)	187

Rich source of calcium, folic acid, iron, magnesium, vitamin A

HEALTH LINKS

Anemia, p. 85; The body's defenses, p. 89

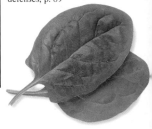

❖ SWISS ONION SOUP ❖

INGREDIENTS

2 tbsp extra-virgin olive oil or canola oil

1lb 2oz (500g) onions, finely sliced

½ garlic clove, crushed

½ tsp brown sugar

4½ cups (1 liter) meat or vegetable stock

freshly ground black pepper

sea salt

4 slices whole-wheat bread

¼ cup (25g) freshly grated Gruyère or Parmesan

1 cup (25g) chopped fresh parsley

⅔ cup (150ml) red wine, optional

This lighter version of the traditional French recipe helps you enjoy a good helping of onions, with their wide-ranging health benefits.

1 In a large, heavy-bottomed pan, heat the oil and add the onions. They should make a thick layer. Stir, then cook uncovered over low heat for about 30 minutes. Stir occasionally to prevent sticking and burning.

2 When the onions are golden and translucent, add the garlic and sugar. Meanwhile, bring the stock to a boil in a saucepan. Pour the boiling stock over the onions, stir well, and when bubbling, lower the heat and simmer, covered, for 20–30 minutes. Season to taste.

3 Place a piece of bread sprinkled with cheese and parsley in each warmed bowl. Heat the soup and add the wine, if using. Pour the soup over and serve.

NUTRITIONAL INFORMATION

Amount per serving

Calories (kcal)	220
Total fat (g)	11
% of calories	44
Sat. fat (g)	3
% of calories	12
Cholesterol (mg)	6
Total carb. (g)	25
Starch (g)	14
Fiber (g)	4
Protein (g)	7
Sodium (mg)	267

HEALTH LINKS

Respiratory infections, p. 76
Gastroenteritis, p. 79
Circulation, pp. 82–5

VARIATIONS

◆ *For a stronger-flavored soup, use 3 cloves of garlic, a full-bodied red wine, and whole-grain garlic bread.*

◆ *Replace the cheese with chopped fresh herbs.*

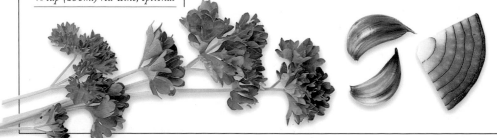

❖ WATERCRESS SOUP ❖

INGREDIENTS

1 tbsp extra-virgin olive oil or butter
1 bunch scallions or 1 leek, finely chopped
1 medium or 2 small potatoes, roughly chopped
4½ cups (1 liter) water or meat or vegetable stock
3 bunches watercress
⅓ cup (75ml) sour cream
pinch of ground nutmeg
freshly ground black pepper
sea salt

This version has a fresher flavor than others and retains the maximum amount of vitamins from the watercress because it is cooked so briefly.

1 In a large saucepan, heat the oil or butter. Add the scallions or leek and cook over low heat until tender, about 10 minutes.

2 Add the potatoes and the water or stock. Bring to a boil, reduce the heat, and simmer, covered, for 10 minutes.

3 Wash, drain, and roughly chop the watercress. Add it to the pan and return to the boil for 2 minutes. Turn off the heat and let stand for 5 minutes.

4 In a blender or food processor, purée the soup and return it to the pan. Stir in the sour cream. Add the nutmeg and season to taste. Reheat gently, do not boil, before serving.

NUTRITIONAL INFORMATION

Amount per serving

Calories (kcal)	120
Total fat (g)	9
% of calories	64
Sat. fat (g)	3
% of calories	24
Cholesterol (mg)	11
Total carb. (g)	7
Starch (g)	5
Fiber (g)	2
Protein (g)	4
Sodium (mg)	49

Rich source of carotenes, folic acid, iron

HEALTH LINKS

Heart health, pp. 82–5
Anemia, p. 85
The body's defenses, p. 89

❖ VEGETABLE CHOWDER ❖

INGREDIENTS

2 tsp extra-virgin olive oil or canola oil
1 tbsp butter
2 onions, finely chopped
1 celery stalk, finely chopped
½ lb (200g) winter squash, peeled, seeded, and diced
⅓ lb (150g) carrots, cut into fat matchsticks
⅓ lb (175g) potatoes, diced
2¼ cups (500ml) vegetable stock
1 bay leaf
⅓ lb (150g) broccoli florets
¼ lb (100g) corn or peas or green beans
2 tomatoes, peeled, seeded, and chopped, optional
2¼ cups (500ml) low-fat milk
3 tbsp chopped fresh herbs, such as basil, oregano, fennel, dill, and parsley, either singly or mixed
freshly ground black pepper
sea salt

This beautiful soup is lighter in taste and texture than traditional chowder. It combines the health bonus of carrots, celery, broccoli, winter squash, and tomatoes. Serves 6

1 Heat the oil and butter in a large pan, add the onions, and stir until sizzling. Adjust the heat to very low and cook for 10 minutes, stirring occasionally, until the onions are soft and translucent.

2 Add the celery, winter squash, carrots, and potatoes. Heat until sizzling, reduce the heat, and cook for 5 minutes longer, stirring occasionally.

3 Add the stock and the bay leaf, bring to a boil, and simmer, covered, for 7–8 minutes, until the potatoes are almost cooked.

4 Add the broccoli, corn (or peas or beans), and tomatoes, if using. Return to a boil and cook vigorously for 3–4 minutes, or until the broccoli is just tender.

5 Stir in the milk and herbs, season to taste, and serve.

NUTRITIONAL INFORMATION

Amount per serving

Calories (k/cal)	188
Total fat (g)	9
% of calories	44
Sat. fat (g)	3
% of calories	14
Cholesterol (mg)	12
Total carb. (g)	21
Starch (g)	10
Fiber (g)	3
Protein (g)	6
Sodium (mg)	81

Rich source of antioxidants, calcium, phosphorus, potassium

HEALTH LINKS

Heart health, pp. 82–5
The body's defenses, p. 89

VARIATION

◆ *To make seafood chowder, add ⅓ lb (150g) mussels or peeled shrimp with the broccoli.*

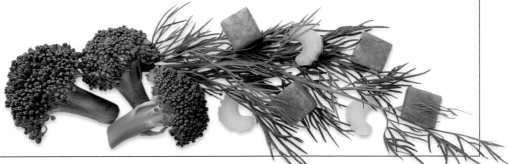

APPETIZERS

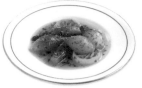

WE EAT APPETIZERS when our appetite is sharpest. As their name suggests, appetizers help create a sense of anticipation for the meal ahead. They also provide an ideal opportunity to enjoy a generous helping of the most valuable foods, such as raw or lightly cooked vegetables and fruits. These can take the edge off your appetite, while their color, crunchy texture, and aroma stimulate the digestive system, preparing it for what is to come. Classic cuisines from many countries have long recognized this: vegetables, such as peppers, fennel, onions, asparagus, and artichokes, are featured in a wide variety of interesting and traditional first courses, ranging from everyday dishes to recipes for special occasions. If you plan a light salad or vegetable main course, you may wish to start with a first course made from foods that are complementary in nutritional value, such as herring or chicken liver; even a small, appetizer-sized portion of these supply a high level of nutrients. This makes a more varied, substantial, and enjoyably balanced meal.

WARM WALNUT DIP WITH GRILLED VEGETABLES
Colorful and appealing, this delicious appetizer is a good way to introduce more vegetables into a meal.

The dip provides essential fatty acids from the walnuts

Sweet potatoes are outstandingly high in vitamin E and beta-carotene

Red peppers are rich in vitamin C, which helps the absorption of iron from the meal

Fennel helps digestion

❖ WARM WALNUT DIP WITH GRILLED VEGETABLES ❖

INGREDIENTS

½ cup (75g) walnut halves

1 cup (200ml) creamy low-fat plain yogurt with active cultures

1 egg white

3 tbsp freshly grated Parmesan

½ garlic clove, crushed

pinch of paprika

2–3 drops chili sauce or 1 tbsp finely chopped fresh herbs

freshly ground black pepper

sea salt

1 fennel bulb, cut into thin segments from the top to the base

1 small sweet potato, thinly sliced

¾ lb (300g) winter squash, peeled, seeded, and thinly sliced

2 tsp extra-virgin olive oil

2 red, orange, or yellow bell peppers, cored, seeded, and cut into 1 inch (2.5cm) strips

2 zucchini, cut into 4 inch (10cm) lengths and quartered

6oz (170g) whole-wheat bread, to serve

Make use of the rich taste of walnuts to tempt the appetite for lightly grilled vegetables, with their important protective properties. Serves 6.

1 Using a food processor or an electric coffee grinder, grind the walnuts into a coarse flour. If any large pieces remain, they add to the texture of the dip.
2 Mix well with the yogurt, egg white, Parmesan, garlic, and paprika. Add the chili sauce or fresh herbs. The chili sauce makes a piquant dip, while fresh herbs, such as dill, basil, parsley, and mint, give a more delicate, aromatic flavor.
3 Pour the mixture into a saucepan and heat gently for 1–3 minutes. Do not boil. The egg white prevents the yogurt from separating when heated. Remove from the heat and season to taste with pepper and salt.
4 To grill the vegetables, heat a small brazier, such as a Japanese hibachi, a broiler, or a cast-iron skillet. Brush the fennel, sweet potato, and winter squash slices lightly with the olive oil. There is no need to brush the bell peppers and zucchini with oil.
5 Cook the vegetables until they just begin to turn brown in places but are still crunchy, 5–10 minutes. The bell peppers and zucchini will cook faster than the other vegetables.
6 Grill a few very thick slices of bread until crisp and then cut into fingers.
7 Serve the dip warm, surrounded by the grilled vegetables and bread.

NUTRITIONAL INFORMATION

Amount per serving
Calories (kcal) — 427
Total fat (g) — 28
% of calories — 58
 Sat. fat (g) — 6
 % of calories — 13
Cholesterol (mg) — 21
Total carb. (g) — 30
 Starch (g) — 16
Fiber (g) — 7
Protein (g) — 16
Sodium (mg) — 305

Rich source of beta-carotene, calcium, folic acid, magnesium, phosphorus, potassium, vitamins C and E, zinc

HEALTH LINKS

Circulation and heart health, pp. 82–5
The body's defenses, p. 89

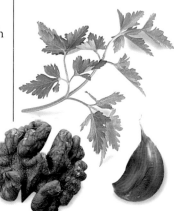

❖ ASPARAGUS WITH PARMESAN & NUTMEG ❖

INGREDIENTS

2 bundles fresh green asparagus

⅓ cup (40g) freshly grated Parmesan

pinch of freshly grated nutmeg

VARIATIONS

◆ Serve hot, with a lightly boiled or poached egg per person in which to dip the spears, or warm with a vinaigrette.

Green asparagus is just as delicious as the more expensive fatter white spears and contains more carotenes and vitamin C.

1 Bring 2½ inches (6cm) water to a boil in the bottom of a steamer, or a specially designed asparagus steamer.
2 Cut any tough ends off the asparagus spears. Remove any rubber bands from the asparagus bundles, rinse, and replace with kitchen string to keep them intact. Steam for 5–10 minutes, or until the bases are tender.
3 Lift out the bundles by hooking a fork through the string. Allow to drain briefly, then place on a warmed, round serving dish. Cut away the string and fan the asparagus spears into a circle.
4 Sprinkle Parmesan over the middle of the spears, leaving the ends and tips clear. Follow with a grating of nutmeg. Serve immediately with finger bowls.

NUTRITIONAL INFORMATION

Amount per serving
Calories (kcal) — 76
Total fat (g) — 4
% of calories — 48
 Sat. fat (g) — 2
 % of calories — 26
Cholesterol (mg) — 10
Total carb. (g) — 3
 Starch (g) — trace
Fiber (g) — 2
Protein (g) — 8
Sodium (mg) — 110

Rich source of folic acid, vitamin C

HEALTH LINKS

Indigestion, p. 78
Kidney function, p. 92

❖ Dill Marinated Herrings ❖

Ingredients

½ cup (140ml) dry sherry

½ cup (140ml)
white wine vinegar

2 tbsp Worcestershire sauce

1 tbsp light brown sugar

¼ cup (15g) chopped fresh dill

2 tbsp sour cream

4 herring fillets, skinned

½ cup (140ml) low-fat plain
yogurt with active cultures

11oz (320g) pumpernickel bread

Marinating lightens the taste of oily fish. This is an ideal appetizer to balance a light main course and also helps iron and zinc absorption, see p. 25.

1 In a medium saucepan, heat the sherry, vinegar, Worcestershire sauce, and sugar and bring to a boil.
2 Remove from the heat and refrigerate for about 10 minutes. Add the dill and sour cream.
3 Cut the herring fillets across into strips about 2 inches (5cm) wide, and place in a glass dish. Pour over the marinade and refrigerate, covered, for at least 48 hours.
4 Stir in the yogurt and serve with slices of pumpernickel bread.

Nutritional Information

Amount per serving	
Calories (kcal)	463
Total fat (g)	16
% of calories	32
Sat. fat (g)	5
% of calories	9
Cholesterol (mg)	56
Total carb. (g)	45
Starch (g)	35
Fiber (g)	4
Protein (g)	27
Sodium (mg)	718

Rich source of calcium, essential fatty acids, iron, selenium, vitamin D

Health Links

Rheumatoid arthritis, p. 81; Heart health, pp. 82–5; Psoriasis, p. 88

❖ Lemon Sardine Pate ❖

Ingredients

2 x 4oz (120g) cans whole
sardines in oil

½ lb (225g) low-fat plain
fromage frais or soft cheese

juice of 2 lemons

freshly ground black pepper

Variation

♦ Replace the sardines with either canned kippers or smoked mackerel, or 2 large fillets of each.

The simplest of fish pâtés, this version is scrumptious on toast or pita and makes a substantial first course with all the benefits of oily fish.

1 Drain the sardines thoroughly. Reserve the oil for use in a salad dressing. Use within 1 week.
2 Mash the fish well with a fork, then mix in the fromage frais or soft cheese. Add the lemon juice and pepper to taste. Chill until ready to serve.

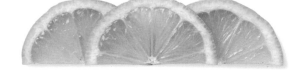

Nutritional Information

Amount per serving	
Calories (kcal)	144
Total fat (g)	7
% of calories	45
Sat. fat (g)	2
% of calories	9
Cholesterol (mg)	33
Total carb. (g)	4
Starch (g)	0
Fiber (g)	trace
Protein (g)	16
Sodium (mg)	244

Rich source of calcium, essential fatty acids, selenium, vitamins B12 and D

Health Links

Osteoporosis, p. 80; Circulation and heart health, pp. 82–5; Psoriasis, p. 88

❖ Chicken Liver & Vermouth Pate ❖

Ingredients

2 tbsp olive oil

1 onion, finely chopped

¾ lb (400g) chicken livers

1 garlic clove, crushed

1 tbsp vermouth

2 tbsp dry red wine or stock

2 tbsp chopped mixed fresh herbs,
such as thyme and marjoram

¼ lb (100g) low-fat soft cheese

freshly ground black pepper

sea salt

Lower in fat than most pâté recipes, this smooth version gives liver a wider appeal.

1 In a heavy-bottomed saucepan, heat the oil, add the onion, and cook uncovered over low heat for 12 minutes, stirring occasionally, until the onion is translucent.
2 Remove any yellow or green parts from the chicken livers and cut each liver into 3 or 4 pieces.
3 Add the liver and garlic to the onions and cook over low heat, stirring often, for 5–6 minutes, or until the liver is lightly cooked through. Do not overcook the liver.
4 Purée the mixture in a blender or food processor, with the vermouth, wine or stock, and the fresh herbs.
5 Return to the pan, mix in the soft cheese, and season to taste. Chill in a serving dish until ready to serve.

Nutritional Information

Amount per serving	
Calories (kcal)	261
Total fat (g)	15
% of calories	53
Sat. fat (g)	4
% of calories	14
Cholesterol (mg)	380
Total carb. (g)	6
Starch (g)	1
Fiber (g)	trace
Protein (g)	23
Sodium (mg)	214

Rich source of folic acid, iron, B vitamins, especially B12, zinc

Health Links

Anemia, p. 85;
The body's defenses, p. 89

❖ ONIONS A LA GRECQUE ❖

This is a very mellow way to eat onions and parsley with the added bonus of garlic and lemon. To balance the oil in the dish, serve it with bread.

INGREDIENTS

1 lemon, plus 4 tsp lemon juice
½ cup (100ml) water
4 tbsp olive oil
3 tbsp dry white wine
1 garlic clove, halved, optional
½ tsp crushed coriander seeds
½ tsp peppercorns, any color
1 bay leaf
1lb 2oz (500g) small onions and/or shallots, preferably red-skinned
sea salt
½ cup (15g) chopped fresh parsley

1 Cut the lemon into 4 thick slices, then cut each slice in half. Remove any seeds.
2 In a saucepan, put the water, oil, wine, half-slices of lemon, 4 teaspoons lemon juice, garlic if using, coriander seeds, peppercorns, and the bay leaf. Bring to a boil. Reduce the heat, cover, and simmer for 10 minutes.
3 Add the onions. Return to a boil, cover, and simmer, stirring occasionally, for about 20 minutes, until the onions are tender but not limp.
4 Remove the onions and lemon slices with a slotted spoon and place them in a serving dish.
5 Boil the liquid uncovered until it is reduced to about half. Taste and adjust the seasoning. Pour over the onions and lemons and let cool. Serve warm or cold, thickly strewn with the chopped parsley, and accompanied by whole-grain bread.

NUTRITIONAL INFORMATION

Amount per serving

Calories (kcal)	194
Total fat (g)	15
% of calories	72
Sat. fat (g)	2
% of calories	10
Cholesterol (mg)	0
Total carb. (g)	11
Starch (g)	trace
Fiber (g)	2
Protein (g)	2
Sodium (mg)	7

Rich source of vitamin C

HEALTH LINKS

Respiratory infections, p. 76
Circulation and heart health, pp. 82–5

VARIATION

◆ *Fennel à la Grecque: Replace the onions with 2 large fennel bulbs cut into ½ inch (1cm) wide segments from the top to the base. Cook for 15 minutes.*

SALADS

A REPERTOIRE OF SALADS based on a wide range of ingredients is the best antidote to the still-common prejudice against cold main courses. Many people tend to be put off by traditional images of plates piled high with lettuce or cabbage, but salads can be based on so many different foods that everyone can find ingredients and combinations they enjoy. There are more than a hundred choices of lettuce and salad greens, and in addition, cooked vegetables, fruit, grains, nuts and seeds, seaweed, and legumes all have salad potential, encouraging people to eat salads more often and in larger helpings. To dispel any lingering chilly image of a salad-based meal, it also helps to choose salads that include warm or more filling ingredients such as pasta or bulgur wheat, or to team salads with a bowl of steaming, hearty soup. People who eat salads with healthy regularity may want to consider using at least some lower-fat dressings, see pp. 140–41. Conventional dressings often have more fat and calories than the salads they accompany.

MUNKAZINA WATERCRESS SALAD
Combining orange, onion, and watercress gives a sparkling sweet-and-tangy mix of flavors and colors, signs of a wide combination of health benefits.

Onions help counter any blood-clotting tendency after eating fatty foods

Oranges are a reliable source of vitamin C

Watercress is rich in folic acid, vitamin C, and iron

❖ MUNKAZINA SALAD ❖

Popular throughout North Africa, this tangy salad provides the benefits of oranges and onions.

1 Slice the oranges across into thin rounds and spread them over a serving dish.
2 Arrange the onion slices and olives on top.
3 Add the dressing, garnish with a sprinkle of paprika, and serve.

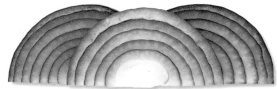

INGREDIENTS

4 medium oranges, peeled

1 red onion, thinly sliced

handful of pitted black olives

pinch of paprika, to garnish

For the dressing

Use a vinaigrette or Yogurt & Mint Dressing, p. 141

VARIATION

◆ *Munkazina Watercress Salad: Add 1 bunch watercress.*

NUTRITIONAL INFORMATION

Amount per serving

Calories (kcal)	112
Total fat (g)	2
% of calories	16
Sat. fat (g)	1
% of calories	3
Cholesterol (mg)	1
Total carb. (g)	21
Starch (g)	trace
Fiber (g)	4
Protein (g)	4
Sodium (mg)	342

Rich source of vitamin C

HEALTH LINKS

Respiratory infections, p. 76
The body's defenses, p. 89

❖ ARTICHOKE HEART SALAD ❖

Artichokes blend beautifully in color and flavor with eggs, lettuce, and shellfish to make an easily digested warm salad or appetizer, or a light meal for 2.

1 If using fresh artichokes, bring a large pan of water to a boil with the wine vinegar. Trim the stems from the artichokes. Immerse them in the boiling water and cook gently for about 35 minutes. If using canned artichoke hearts, drain and set them aside.
2 Meanwhile, boil the eggs for 8 minutes, then let them stand in cold water until cool enough to handle. Drain and peel them carefully; they should barely be hard.
3 Bring a small saucepan of water to a boil, add the shrimp, and cook for 3 minutes. Drain and let cool, then toss with the shredded lettuce.
4 Drain the fresh artichokes. Remove the tough outer leaves and scrape out the hairy "choke" from each one. Keep the softer, central leaves for use in other dishes.
5 Make a circle of the shredded lettuce and shrimp mixture on each plate. Place on it either a quartered fresh artichoke heart, or 2 halved, canned artichoke hearts. Cut the eggs across and place one half in the center of each portion of artichoke heart. Drizzle with dressing and serve.

INGREDIENTS

4 large globe artichokes or 1 x 14oz (400g) can or jar artichoke hearts

1 tbsp wine vinegar

2 eggs

¼ lb (100g) shrimp, peeled weight

1 head lettuce or other salad greens, such as escarole, shredded

For the dressing

Use a vinaigrette or Yogurt & Mint Dressing, p. 141, replacing the mint with extra chives or parsley if you prefer

NUTRITIONAL INFORMATION

Amount per serving

Calories (kcal)	150
Total fat (g)	4
% of calories	25
Sat. fat (g)	1
% of calories	8
Cholesterol (mg)	147
Total carb. (g)	14
Starch (g)	trace
Fiber (g)	1
Protein (g)	19
Sodium (mg)	248

Rich source of calcium, copper, folic acid, iron, magnesium, phosphorus, potassium, vitamin B12, zinc

HEALTH LINKS

Digestion, pp. 78–9; Gallstones, p. 79; Anemia, p. 85, Sleep problems, p. 93

VARIATION

◆ *Replace the shrimp with a grilled red pepper, cut into strips.*

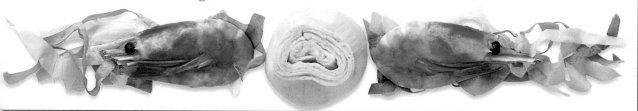

❖ ARAME, BROCCOLI & WALNUT SALAD ❖

INGREDIENTS

1oz (30g) arame, dry weight

2 carrots, cut into matchsticks

½ lb (225g) broccoli florets

For the dressing

¼ cup (25g) walnut pieces, lightly toasted and chopped

2 tsp sweet rice vinegar

1 tbsp unrefined sunflower oil and sesame oil, mixed

1 tbsp light soy sauce

3 tbsp unsweetened apple juice

Slim, juicy strands of Japanese arame seaweed combine well with broccoli, carrots, and a walnut dressing in color, taste, texture, and health value.

1 Rinse the arame in a sieve under running water, then place the sieve in a deep bowl. Cover the arame with cold water and soak for 5–6 minutes to soften it. Lift out the sieve and drain the arame.

2 Fill a saucepan with water to a depth of 1 inch (2.5cm) and bring to a boil. Add the carrots and cook for 3–4 minutes. Add the broccoli and cook for 4 more minutes, then drain.

3 In a serving bowl, mix all the dressing ingredients.

4 Add the arame and vegetables to the dressing, toss well, and serve.

NUTRITIONAL INFORMATION

Amount per serving

Calories (kcal)	125
Total fat (g)	9
% of calories	64
Sat. fat (g)	1
% of calories	7
Cholesterol (mg)	0
Total carb. (g)	7
Starch (g)	trace
Fiber (g)	6
Protein (g)	5
Sodium (mg)	474

Rich source of antioxidants, folic acid

HEALTH LINK

Heart health, pp. 82–5

❖ WALDORF SALAD ❖

INGREDIENTS

squeeze of lemon or orange juice

¾ lb (350g) apples, preferably red-skinned

¾ lb (350g) celery, chopped into ½ inch (1cm) thick pieces

¼ cup (25g) walnut halves, roughly chopped

2 tbsp chopped fresh chives, parsley, fennel, or dill, to garnish

For the dressing

Use Yogurt & Mint Dressing, p. 141

A classic fall and winter salad, this recipe combines the health benefits of apples, celery, and walnuts. Red-skinned apples are prettiest for this salad.

1 Squeeze the citrus juice into a serving bowl.

2 Scrub the apples with warm, soapy water and rinse, unless organic, in which case rinse them in cold water. Dry the apples and dice them into the bowl. Toss well with the citrus juice to prevent discoloration.

3 Stir in the celery and walnuts.

4 Add the dressing and toss gently to coat the salad ingredients well.

5 Garnish with the fresh herbs and serve immediately. If the salad needs to be made ahead, cover with plastic wrap and refrigerate, but allow it to reach room temperature before serving. Use the same day.

NUTRITIONAL INFORMATION

Amount per serving

Calories (kcal)	97
Total fat (g)	5
% of calories	45
Sat. fat (g)	1
% of calories	5
Cholesterol (mg)	1
Total carb. (g)	11
Starch (g)	trace
Fiber (g)	3
Protein (g)	3
Sodium (mg)	77

Rich source of vitamin C

HEALTH LINKS

Constipation, p. 78
Heart health, pp. 82–5
Fluid retention, p. 84

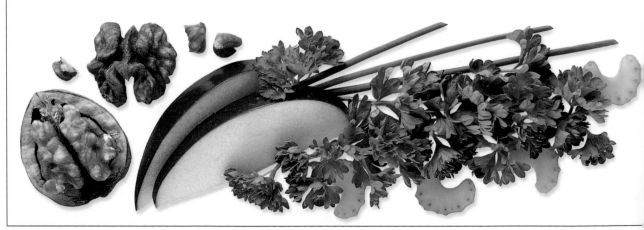

❖ SUMMER HERB SALAD ❖

Lavish use of fresh herbs is the key to this quick and simple warm salad, which is one of the best ways to use whole-wheat pasta, with its superior health value.

1 Bring a large saucepan of water to a boil, add the pasta, and cook vigorously, uncovered, for 12–14 minutes, or until just tender.
2 Meanwhile, chop half the herbs fine, the other half more roughly. Rub them between your fingers into a serving bowl to release their flavor. Stir in the oil.
3 Drain the pasta, leaving a little water on it. Stir into the bowl of herbs and toss well. Let stand for about 10 minutes and serve warm.

INGREDIENTS

½ lb (250g) whole-wheat pasta

1¼ oz (35g) any mixture of fresh herbs, such as parsley, chives, oregano, basil, dill, tarragon, mint, marjoram, fennel, chervil, and cilantro. Use only a few leaves of stronger-flavored herbs, such as rosemary or sage, to prevent their flavor from overwhelming the salad.

2 tbsp extra-virgin olive oil

NUTRITIONAL INFORMATION

Amount per serving

Calories (kcal)	272
Total fat (g)	9
% of calories	30
Sat. fat (g)	1
% of calories	4
Cholesterol (mg)	0
Total carb. (g)	42
Starch (g)	39
Fiber (g)	6
Protein (g)	9
Sodium (mg)	83

Rich source of copper, zinc

HEALTH LINKS

Constipation, p. 78
Heart health, pp. 82–5

❖ SHIRO AE SALAD ❖

Translating as "white salad," this Japanese dish is substantial in character. The tofu and sesame dressing is an especially good source of calcium.

1 Put the mushrooms in a small, heatproof bowl, cover with boiling water, and soak until soft, about 30 minutes. Strain and slice them very thin.
2 Meanwhile, in a saucepan, bring the soy sauce and water to a boil. Add the mirin, the mushrooms, carrots, and green beans. Cook, covered, on medium-high heat for 5 minutes; strain and set aside.
3 To make the dressing, first drain the tofu in a sieve retaining the liquid for stock. Mash the tofu with a fork.
4 Heat an ungreased, heavy-bottomed skillet, add the sesame seeds, and cook over low heat for 3–4 minutes, shaking often, until they start to turn golden. Remove from the heat and crush them with a mortar and pestle.
5 In a blender or food processor, purée the tofu with the sesame seeds, soy sauce, and mirin.
6 In a serving bowl, toss the arame, cucumber, or radish with the warm vegetables. Stir in the tofu dressing. Divide among salad plates, sprinkle crisp nori flakes on top of each salad, and serve.

INGREDIENTS

4 dried shiitake or cepe mushrooms

2 tsp light soy sauce

1¼ cups (300ml) water

1 tbsp mirin, or 1 tbsp sake plus 1 tsp sugar

⅓ lb (150g) carrots, cut into long, very thin strips

⅓ lb (150g) green beans, cut into long, very thin strips

⅓ lb (150g) soaked arame, or cucumber, cut into long, very thin strips, or shredded daikon

For the dressing

½ lb (200g) soft tofu

2 tbsp sesame seeds

2 tbsp light soy sauce

1 tbsp mirin, or 1 tbsp sake plus 1 tsp sugar

2 tsp (5g) nori flakes or a shredded nori sheet, to garnish

NUTRITIONAL INFORMATION

Amount per serving

Calories (kcal)	140
Total fat (g)	7
% of calories	43
Sat. fat (g)	1
% of calories	6
Cholesterol (mg)	0
Total carb. (g)	12
Starch (g)	1
Fiber (g)	4
Protein (g)	8
Sodium (mg)	600

Rich source of calcium, carotenes, phosphorus

HEALTH LINK

Menopause, p. 87

VARIATION

♦ *Replace the green beans and carrots with other vegetables that are colorful and crisp in texture, like broccoli florets and red pepper, or scallions and corn.*

❖ SUNFLOWER GREEN SALAD ❖

INGREDIENTS

¼ cup (50g) sunflower seeds

1 head lettuce or mixed salad greens

¼ cup (25g) freshly grated Parmesan

For the dressing

Use Honey & Mustard Dressing, p. 140, omitting the sea salt

Sunflower seeds are one of the most effective ways to get more vitamin E and add an interesting crunch and flavor to salad greens.

1 Put the sunflower seeds in an ungreased skillet and heat gently for a few minutes, shaking often, to bring out their flavor.
2 In a serving bowl, mix together the hot seeds, salad greens, and Parmesan. Add the dressing, toss well, and serve.

NUTRITIONAL INFORMATION

Amount per serving
Calories (kcal)	14
Total fat (g)	1
% of calories	6
Sat. fat (g)	
% of calories	1
Cholesterol (mg)	
Total carb. (g)	0
Starch (g)	2
Fiber (g)	
Protein (g)	
Sodium (mg)	9

Rich source of folic acid, vitamin E

HEALTH LINKS

Heart health, pp. 82–5
The body's defenses, p. 89

❖ SLAW SALAD ❖

INGREDIENTS

½ lb (225g) cabbage, preferably green or bok choi, finely shredded

¼ lb (150g) carrots, coarsely grated

1 red-skinned apple, well scrubbed and diced

¼ cup (40g) raisins

For the dressing

Use Honey & Mustard Dressing, p. 140

A freshly prepared slaw salad, served with bread or a baked potato, is a simple, enjoyable way to improve your intake of vegetables and fiber.

1 Combine the ingredients in a large bowl.
2 Add the dressing and toss gently to coat the salad well. Serve at once or chill until ready to use. Eat the same day the salad is prepared.

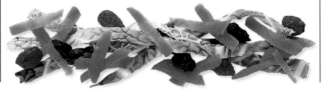

NUTRITIONAL INFORMATION

Amount per serving
Calories (kcal)	9
Total fat (g)	
% of calories	2
Sat. fat (g)	
% of calories	
Cholesterol (mg)	
Total carb. (g)	1
Starch (g)	trace
Fiber (g)	
Protein (g)	
Sodium (mg)	4

Rich source of antioxidants

HEALTH LINKS

Heart health, pp. 82–5
The body's defenses, p. 89

❖ TOMATO & WHEAT GERM SALAD ❖

INGREDIENTS

1¼ lb (600g) fresh tomatoes, thickly sliced

¾ cup (100g) wheat germ

½ cup (50g) golden linseed, crushed

½ cup (100ml) low-fat plain yogurt

3 tbsp rice vinegar

½ cup (120ml) skim milk

3 tbsp chopped fresh herbs, such as basil, parsley, chives, and oregano

1 tsp honey, optional

Linseed and wheat germ add a crunchy sweetness to this salad, and this dish helps improve your intake of vitamin E and omega-3 fatty acids.

1 Place the tomato slices in a large bowl.
2 Add the remaining ingredients and toss gently to coat the salad well. Taste and add the honey, if desired.
3 Serve at once.

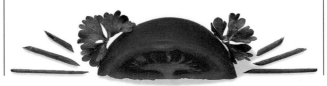

NUTRITIONAL INFORMATION

Amount per serving
Calories (kcal)	21
Total fat (g)	1
% of calories	4
Sat. fat (g)	
% of calories	
Cholesterol (mg)	
Total carb. (g)	2
Starch (g)	
Fiber (g)	0
Protein (g)	
Sodium (mg)	5

Rich source of omega-3 fatty acids, potassium, vitamin E

HEALTH LINKS

Heart health, pp. 82–5
Menopause, p. 87

❖ TABBOULEH ❖

INGREDIENTS

½ cup (75g) bulgur wheat
1–2 cups (50–75g) chopped fresh parsley
4–5 scallions, finely chopped
3 sprigs fresh mint, finely chopped
1 garlic clove, crushed
1 tbsp extra-virgin olive oil
juice of 1 lemon
2–3 fresh tomatoes, peeled and diced, optional
freshly ground black pepper
sea salt

This is a classic Middle Eastern salad. It features parsley as a main ingredient, in large enough quantities to take full advantage of its health benefits.

1 Rinse the bulgur wheat grains in a large sieve under cold running water. Place the sieve in a bowl and cover with boiling water, ensuring the grains are covered.

2 Let stand for 20 minutes, until the grains have absorbed enough water to become tender.

3 Meanwhile, in a serving bowl, mix all the other ingredients except the pepper and salt.

4 Take out the sieve and press down on the grains, to remove any excess water.

5 Add the grains to the other ingredients, toss well, and season to taste. Let the mixture stand for at least 15 minutes before serving.

NUTRITIONAL INFORMATION

Amount per serving	
Calories (kcal)	117
Total fat (g)	4
% of calories	35
Sat. fat (g)	1
% of calories	4
Cholesterol (mg)	0
Total carb. (g)	17
Starch (g)	16
Fiber (g)	1
Protein (g)	3
Sodium (mg)	11
Rich source of vitamin C	

HEALTH LINKS

Anemia, p. 85
The body's defenses, p. 89
Kidney function, p. 92

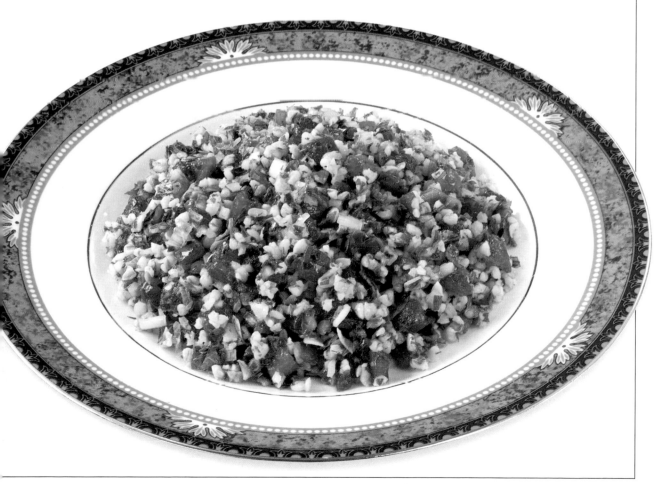

MAIN COURSES

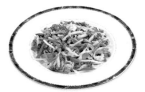

TODAY'S BEST MAIN COURSES do not rely on slabs of meat or fish, but on smaller amounts of meat or fish with an interesting flavor, which complements a generous serving of rice, bread, pasta, or other starchy foods. The meat and fish dishes in this section are designed to be eaten in this style. Fish is a food highly suited to modern needs: whether low-fat shellfish or oily fish rich in omega-3 fatty acids, we benefit from eating fish more often, and it is also one of the quickest foods to cook. While poultry has the attraction of a low fat level, lean red mea[t] has merits too, especially for young people with high iron needs. One dish main courses feature starch[y] foods or vegetables as the mai[n] ingredient, enhanced by a variety o[f] spices and flavorings drawn from tradition[al] recipes around the world. Whether or not the[y] include meat or fish, these dishes provid[e] enough protein for a main course. Dishes suc[h] as risottos, pilafs, or stir-fries show the variet[y] of main courses that can be made with little o[r] no meat or fish, and how good they can taste.

GREEK FISH STEW
This quick fish casserole is a tasty way to eat more oily fish, which provide omega-3 fatty acids and vitamin E.

Mussels are a rich source of iron

Tomatoes supply antioxidants

Shrimp is a good source of zinc an[d] vitamin E

❖ GREEK FISH STEW ❖

INGREDIENTS

1 tbsp extra-virgin olive oil
1 onion or 6 shallots, finely chopped
1 large or 2 small garlic cloves, finely chopped
1lb 2oz (500g) fresh tomatoes, peeled and roughly chopped
½ cup (100ml) dry white wine
½ cup (100ml) water
1½ lb (700g) boneless fish, such as swordfish or sea trout, cut into chunks, and shellfish, such as shrimp and mussels, or a mixture of these seafoods
½ bunch chopped fresh parsley
2 tbsp chopped fresh fennel fronds, optional
juice of 1 lemon
freshly ground black pepper
sea salt

This easy, adaptable fish stew can be made in 15 minutes from scratch. It combines any mixture of white fish, oily fish, and shellfish.

1 In a large skillet, heat the oil and cook the onion and garlic over low heat for 5 minutes, stirring often.
2 Add the tomatoes, wine, and water and cook for 8–10 minutes, until the tomatoes are soft. Do not cook the tomatoes any longer; brief cooking keeps their fresh taste and retains more vitamin C.
3 Add the fish chunks and/or shellfish, return to a boil, and cook over medium heat for 5 minutes, until just tender. Avoid overcooking.
4 Remove from the heat, stir in the parsley, fennel, if using, and lemon juice. Season to taste and serve at once.

NUTRITIONAL INFORMATION

Amount per serving

Calories (kcal)	247
Total fat (g)	8
% of calories	30
Sat. fat (g)	1
% of calories	3
Cholesterol (mg)	171
Total carb. (g)	6
Starch (g)	trace
Fiber (g)	2
Protein (g)	34
Sodium (mg)	235

Rich source of carotenes, iron, phosphorus, potassium, selenium, vitamins B12, C, and E, zinc

HEALTH LINKS

Circulation and heart health, pp. 82–5
The body's defenses, p. 89

❖ MOULES MARINIERE ❖

INGREDIENTS

2 tsp extra-virgin olive oil
1 small onion, finely chopped
1 garlic clove, crushed, optional
1¼ cups (300ml) dry red or white wine
freshly ground black pepper
4lb (1.8kg) fresh mussels
3 tbsp chopped fresh parsley

VARIATION

♦ *Replace the mussels with clams.*

Served with bread, this is a classic, quick meal. All mussels have a high food value, and New Zealand green-lipped mussels may help relieve rheumatoid arthritis.

1 To clean the mussels, scrub the outer shells with a stiff brush and pull out the small strands, known as beards, that stick out of the side of the shell.
2 In a very large saucepan, heat the oil and gently cook the onion and garlic, if using, for about 8 minutes, stirring often.
3 Add the wine and some pepper and bring to a boil. Add the mussels, cover tightly, and steam for 2–3 minutes, shaking the pan often.
4 As soon as the mussels have opened, remove from the heat. Strain, retaining the cooking liquid. Discard any mussels that have not opened.
5 Return the cooking liquid to the pan through a cheesecloth-lined sieve to remove any grit. Reheat and boil for a few minutes.
6 Divide the mussels among the serving bowls. Stir the parsley into the sauce, pour over the mussels, and serve at once.

NUTRITIONAL INFORMATION

Amount per serving

Calories (kcal)	213
Total fat (g)	6
% of calories	25
Sat. fat (g)	1
% of calories	3
Cholesterol (mg)	72
Total carb. (g)	7
Starch (g)	trace
Fiber (g)	1
Protein (g)	21
Sodium (mg)	444

Rich source of copper, folic acid, iron, phosphorus, selenium, vitamin B12, zinc

HEALTH LINKS

Arthritis, p. 81; Anemia, p. 85;
The body's defenses,
p. 89

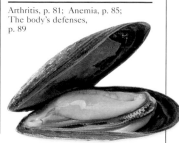

❖ SALMON KEDGEREE ❖

INGREDIENTS

1½ lb (675g) salmon
1 tbsp extra-virgin olive oil
4 cloves
1 cinnamon stick
3 cardamom pods, bruised
1½ cups (250g) long-grain rice, preferably brown basmati
1 onion, finely chopped
1 inch (2.5cm) piece fresh ginger, finely sliced
2 garlic cloves, finely sliced
½ tsp garam masala
½ small red chili pepper, seeded and finely minced, or ½ tsp chili powder
¼ cup (25g) unblanched almonds, chopped into slivers
juice of 1 lemon or lime
2 tbsp raisins, optional
2 hard-boiled eggs, chopped
chopped fresh parsley, to garnish

Mildly hot, Indian-style kedgeree combines no fewer than 7 bonus foods, with a wide range of health benefits, especially for the circulation.

1 Cut the salmon into 1 inch (2.5cm) cubes; set aside.
2 Heat half the oil in a large saucepan. Add the cloves, cinnamon, and cardamom and stir over medium heat for 1 minute. Add the rice and continue stirring for another minute.
3 Add double the volume of water for ordinary long-grain rice or 2½ cups (600ml) for basmati rice and bring to a boil. Stir once, cover, reduce the heat to the lowest setting, and simmer for 20–45 minutes, or until all the water is absorbed.
4 Meanwhile, in another saucepan, heat the remaining oil and gently cook the onion, ginger, and garlic for 5 minutes. Add the garam masala, chili or chili powder, and almonds and cook for 1 minute, stirring often. Add the salmon, sprinkle it with the lemon or lime juice, cover, and cook for about 5 minutes, or until tender.
5 When the rice is cooked, remove the cinnamon and cloves. Add the salmon mixture and the raisins, if using, stirring carefully so that the salmon does not break up.
6 Cook over very low heat, covered, for 15 minutes to allow the flavors to blend. Check the seasoning.
7 Garnish with the chopped eggs and the parsley. Serve at once.

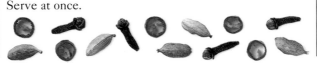

NUTRITIONAL INFORMATION

Amount per serving

Calories (kcal)	685
Total fat (g)	31
% of calories	41
Sat. fat (g)	5
% of calories	7
Cholesterol (mg)	181
Total carb. (g)	62
Starch (g)	54
Fiber (g)	1
Protein (g)	44
Sodium (mg)	126

Rich source of phosphorus, selenium, vitamins B12 and E, zinc

HEALTH LINKS

Respiratory infections, p. 76
Rheumatoid arthritis, p. 81
Circulation and heart health, pp. 82–5

VARIATIONS

◆ *Replace the salmon with smoked haddock or shrimp, either singly or mixed with other shellfish or white fish.*
◆ *Bean Kedgeree: cooked lentils, split peas, or kidney beans can be used in place of fish. Use ¼ cup (60g) dry weight per person, soaked overnight, drained, and cooked in fresh water until tender. Add in step 5, when the rice is cooked.*

❖ SHRIMP IN GREEN TEA ❖

INGREDIENTS

1 tbsp green tea leaves
1 cup (225ml) boiling water
1½ tbsp canola oil
1lb 2oz (500g) fresh or frozen shrimp, peeled or unpeeled as preferred
1 tbsp sake or dry sherry

A delicate Chinese recipe for shrimp, this dish complements other subtle flavors, such as jasmine rice, and brings the benefits of green tea to a main course.

1 Place the tea leaves in a heatproof measuring cup and pour over the boiling water. Let steep for 15 minutes.
2 Heat the oil until very hot. Add the shrimp and sake or sherry and cook over high heat for 1 minute, stirring continuously.
3 Add the tea and about half the tea leaves and cook for another minute.
4 Using a slotted spoon, lift out the shrimp and place them on a warmed serving dish. Keep the heat turned up and reduce the cooking liquid to about ¾ cup (150ml). Pour over the shrimp and serve at once with rice.

NUTRITIONAL INFORMATION

Amount per serving

Calories (kcal)	149
Total fat (g)	6
% of calories	38
Sat. fat (g)	1
% of calories	3
Cholesterol (mg)	244
Total carb. (g)	trace
Starch (g)	0
Fiber (g)	0
Protein (g)	22
Sodium (mg)	238

Rich source of phosphorus, vitamins B12 and E

HEALTH LINKS

Heart health, pp. 82–5
The body's defenses, p. 89

❖ LAMB PASANDA ❖

INGREDIENTS

1 tbsp canola oil
1 large onion, thinly sliced
1lb 2oz (500g) lean lamb, such as neck fillet, cut into cubes
2 garlic cloves, crushed
1 inch (2.5cm) piece fresh ginger, finely grated
½ tsp ground turmeric
2 tsp ground coriander
1 tsp ground cumin
½ tsp nutmeg, freshly grated
large pinch of cayenne
scant 1 cup (200ml) water
½ cup (50g) whole unblanched almonds
1¼ cups (300ml) low-fat plain yogurt
1 tsp garam masala
sea salt

Spicy but not fiery hot, this pale gold lamb dish looks as good as it tastes and includes the benefits of 6 bonus foods.

1 In a large saucepan, heat half the oil and cook the onion, uncovered, for 10 minutes, until softened. Remove the onion with a slotted spoon and set aside.
2 Add the remaining oil to the pan and heat. Add the lamb and cook for a few minutes over medium heat, stirring often, until browned. Add the garlic, ginger, turmeric, coriander, cumin, nutmeg, and cayenne and, when hot, reduce the heat and cook for 2 minutes, stirring often.
3 Return the onion to the pan and add the water. Bring to a boil, reduce the heat and simmer, covered, stirring occasionally, for 30 minutes, or until the meat is tender. Cook uncovered during the last 5 minutes.
4 Meanwhile, to toast the almonds, heat them for 2–3 minutes over low heat in an ungreased skillet. Cut about 10 into slivers for the garnish and grind the remainder in an electric coffee grinder.
5 Remove the lamb from the heat and stir in the yogurt, ground almonds, and garam masala. Season to taste.
6 Garnish with the slivered almonds and serve. If reheating, do not allow the mixture to boil.

NUTRITIONAL INFORMATION

Amount per serving

Calories (kcal)	375
Total fat (g)	23
% of calories	56
Sat. fat (g)	7
% of calories	16
Cholesterol (mg)	102
Total carb. (g)	11
Starch (g)	1
Fiber (g)	2
Protein (g)	34
Sodium (mg)	178

Rich source of calcium, copper, iron, magnesium, phosphorus, vitamins B12 and E, zinc

HEALTH LINKS

Gastroenteritis, p. 79; Circulation and heart health, pp. 82–5

❖ FORTY-CLOVE GARLIC CHICKEN ❖

INGREDIENTS

1 chicken, about 3lb (1.3kg)
1 tbsp extra-virgin olive oil
½ lb (250g) celery, roughly sliced
8 small carrots, well scrubbed
40 garlic cloves (or 30 if large), unpeeled, preferably purple-skinned
½ cup (140ml) dry white wine
2 x 1 inch (2.5cm) thin strips lemon zest
4 x 2 inch (5cm) sprigs fresh thyme
1 tbsp balsamic vinegar, optional
freshly ground black pepper

Thanks to the slow, gentle cooking of the garlic cloves, this recipe is far from overpowering, and you do not have to peel the garlic cloves. Purple garlic is prettiest.

1 Preheat the oven to 375°F/190°C. Cut the chicken in half lengthwise.
2 Heat the oil in a wide, flat, flameproof casserole dish and brown each chicken half over medium-high heat.
3 Reduce the heat and lift out the chicken halves. Add the celery, whole carrots, and garlic. Stir for 2 minutes and then place the chicken halves on top, together with the wine, lemon zest, and 2 sprigs of thyme. Bring to a boil and turn off the heat.
4 To ensure no steam escapes during baking, place a double layer of foil over the casserole dish before gently pressing down the lid. Bake for 1½ hours.
5 Remove the lid, stir in the vinegar, if using, and season to taste. Place the remaining thyme sprigs on top for the garnish and serve.

NUTRITIONAL INFORMATION

Amount per serving

Calories (kcal)	297
Total fat (g)	11
% of calories	33
Sat. fat (g)	3
% of calories	9
Cholesterol (mg)	88
Total carb. (g)	11
Starch (g)	2
Fiber (g)	4
Protein (g)	35
Sodium (mg)	192

Rich source of copper, phosphorus, vitamin A, zinc

HEALTH LINKS

Respiratory infections, p. 76
Gastroenteritis, p. 79
Circulation and heart health, pp. 82–5

❖ GEORGIAN CHICKEN WITH WALNUTS ❖

INGREDIENTS

1 chicken, about 3lb (1.3kg)
2 bay leaves
1 tbsp unrefined sunflower oil
2 onions, finely sliced
1–2 garlic cloves, crushed
1 tsp crushed coriander seeds
¾ cup (100g) walnut halves, roughly crushed
½ lb (200g) plums, pitted
1 tsp sweet cayenne
1 tsp ground cinnamon
large pinch of ground cloves
3 slices whole-wheat bread
juice of ½ pomegranate, or juice of ½ lemon plus ½ tsp honey or sugar
2 tbsp chopped fresh cilantro
freshly ground black pepper
sea salt
2 tbsp chopped fresh mint, to garnish

Walnuts, rather than high-saturate butter or cream, are the basis of a luxurious satsivi sauce that complements chicken, meat, or fish. The fruit in this dish is typical of Central Asian cookery.

1 Cut the chicken into 4 pieces, retaining the carcass. Place the chicken and the carcass in a large saucepan, add the bay leaves, and enough water to cover. Bring to a boil, cover tightly, reduce the heat, and simmer for about 45 minutes.

2 Meanwhile, heat the oil in a large skillet and gently cook the onions for 10 minutes, stirring often. Add the garlic, coriander, and walnuts and cook for 3–4 more minutes. Remove from the heat and set aside.

3 Remove the chicken and strain 1¾ cups (400ml) of the cooking liquid into a small pitcher and refrigerate for about 20 minutes. Then skim off the fat, which will have risen to the surface.

4 To make the satsivi sauce, purée the onion mixture with the skimmed stock, plums, cayenne, cinnamon, cloves, bread, pomegranate or lemon juice, and half the cilantro. Return the mixture to the skillet and add the chicken.

5 Stir and cook gently for 10 minutes. Season to taste. Garnish with the remaining cilantro and the mint and serve.

NUTRITIONAL INFORMATION

Amount per serving

Calories (kcal)	473
Total fat (g)	29
% of calories	54
Sat. fat (g)	4
% of calories	8
Cholesterol (mg)	88
Total carb. (g)	18
Starch (g)	5
Fiber (g)	3
Protein (g)	38
Sodium (mg)	203

Rich source of copper, phosphorus, zinc

HEALTH LINK

Circulation and heart health, pp. 82–5

VARIATION

◆ *Serve this satsivi walnut sauce, hot or cold, separately from the chicken, or with other meat or fish.*

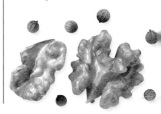

❖ BEEF & CARROT TZIMMES ❖

INGREDIENTS

1lb (400g) beef brisket, boned
2 onions, halved
1 cup (225g) prunes, pitted
4 cloves
1 tsp ground ginger
1¼ cups (300ml) water
1½ lb (700g) carrots, sliced
2 tbsp honey
juice of 1–2 lemons
freshly ground black pepper
sea salt

This spicy-sweet stew, simplified from the traditional Jewish culinary repertoire, is a tasty way to eat more carotene-rich carrots.

1 Trim as much fat from the meat as possible. Heat a large, heavy-bottomed saucepan, put the meat in skin side down, and brown. When some of the fat has melted, turn the meat, browning it on all sides. Add the onions and brown for a few minutes, stirring often.

2 Add the prunes, spices, and water. Bring to a boil, cover tightly, reduce the heat and simmer gently for 1½–2 hours, until the meat is tender.

3 Add the carrots and honey, return to a boil, and cook gently for about 40 minutes, until the carrots are tender. Remove from the heat.

4 Strain off most of the cooking liquid into a saucepan and boil it vigorously for 4–5 minutes, to reduce.

5 Return the reduced cooking liquid to the meat and carrot mixture. Add the lemon juice, season to taste, and serve.

NUTRITIONAL INFORMATION

Amount per serving

Calories (kcal)	376
Total fat (g)	13
% of calories	32
Sat. fat (g)	5
% of calories	12
Cholesterol (mg)	67
Total carb. (g)	44
Starch (g)	1
Fiber (g)	8
Protein (g)	22
Sodium (mg)	118

Rich source of carotenes, iron, phosphorus, potassium, vitamins A and B12, zinc

HEALTH LINKS

Anemia, p. 85;
The body's defenses, p. 89

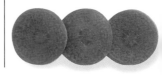

❖ SALMON TERIYAKI ❖

INGREDIENTS

1½ lb (600g) oily fish steaks, such as salmon, mackerel, swordfish, trout, or eel

oil to coat an iron skillet

For the sauce

2 tbsp dark soy sauce

1 tbsp brown sugar

4 tbsp sake

VARIATION

◆ *Use chicken or turkey breast or thigh meat, pork fillet, or beefsteak, cut into thick pieces.*

Teriyaki is a glaze-grill method of cooking that is one of the quickest and easiest ways to give extra flavor to grilled fish or meat, without extra fat.

1 Cut the fish into thick pieces.
2 Lightly brush an iron skillet with the oil and heat under a hot broiler or over a very high heat until very hot but not smoking.
3 Add the fish and broil or fry until cooked through and crisp on both sides.
4 In a bowl, mix the soy sauce with the sugar. Pour the sake over the fish and light it with a match. After the flame dies away, turn up the heat and brush the pieces heavily on both sides with the soy sauce mixture.
5 Cook for 1–2 minutes more, until the sauce becomes sticky. Place the fish on a warmed dish, pour over any remaining sauce, and serve.

NUTRITIONAL INFORMATION

Amount per serving

Calories (kcal)	312
Total fat (g)	19
% of calories	55
Sat. fat (g)	3
% of calories	9
Cholesterol (mg)	75
Total carb. (g)	5
Starch (g)	0
Fiber (g)	0
Protein (g)	31
Sodium (mg)	498

Rich source of niacin, phosphorus, selenium, vitamins B$_6$ and B$_{12}$

HEALTH LINKS

Rheumatoid arthritis, p. 81
Circulation and heart health, pp. 82–5
Psoriasis, p. 88

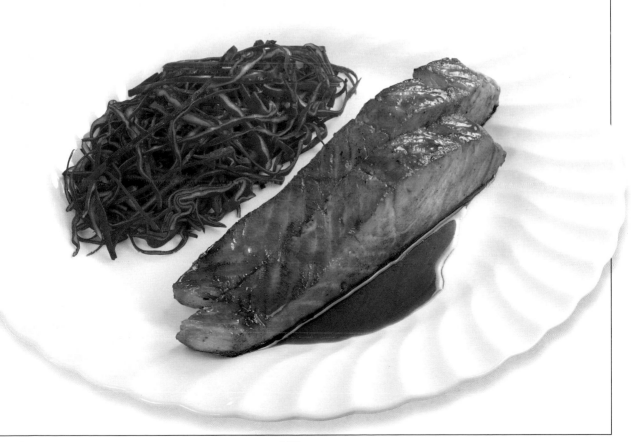

❖ ASPARAGUS FRITTATA ❖

INGREDIENTS

*½ lb (250g) fresh green
asparagus, trimmed*

1 tbsp sunflower oil

*½ lb (55g) freshly grated
Parmesan*

freshly ground black pepper

8 eggs, beaten

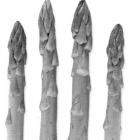

*To help balance the relatively high percentage
of fat in this dish, serve it with plenty of rice,
baked sweet potato, or other starchy food.*

1 Steam or boil the asparagus for 3–5 minutes, or until
barely cooked, and drain. Chop the asparagus into
2 inch (5cm) lengths.
2 In a small, heavy-bottomed skillet, heat half of the
oil and quickly sauté the asparagus for 2–3 minutes
over high heat. Remove and set aside.
3 Mix the Parmesan and pepper into the beaten eggs.
4 Add the remaining oil to the pan and heat. Reduce
the heat and pour in the eggs. After about 1 minute,
add the asparagus. Continue to cook for about 8 minutes
over very low heat.
5 Heat the broiler to moderate. When the bottom of
the frittata is set, place the pan under the broiler for 1–2
minutes, until the top is just set.
6 Slide the frittata onto a plate and serve hot, warm,
or cold, cut into wedges.

NUTRITIONAL INFORMATION

Amount per serving

Calories/(k/cals)	258/1073
Total fat (g)	19
% of calories	68
Sat. fat (g)	6
% of calories	22
Cholesterol. (mg)	399
Total carb. (g)	1
Starch (g)	trace
Fiber (g)	1
Protein (g)	20
Sodium (mg)	291

Rich source of calcium, folic acid, zinc,
phosphorus, vitamins A, B12, and E

HEALTH LINK

Kidney function, p. 92

VARIATION

◆ *Artichoke Frittata: Use ½ lb
(250g) canned artichoke hearts,
drained weight.*

❖ CELERY AMANDINE ❖

INGREDIENTS

*4 small heads green celery,
trimmed and halved lengthwise*

*2 tsp sunflower oil or a mixture
of sunflower oil and butter*

*4 garlic cloves, quartered,
optional*

1¼ cups (300ml) water or stock

*½ cup (60g) freshly grated
Parmesan*

*¾ cup (100g) unblanched
almonds, cut into slivers*

freshly ground black pepper

*Crisp green celery lends its color and flavor
to this light and elegant main course.*

1 Separate the celery stalks and then trim them into
7 inch (18cm) lengths. Place the celery halves in a layer
in the bottom of a wide saucepan or skillet with lid.
2 In another saucepan, heat 1 teaspoon oil or butter.
Add the garlic, if using, and cook for about 2 minutes
over medium heat, stirring often. Add the water or
stock and bring to a boil. Remove from the heat and
pour over the celery halves.
3 Bring the celery and water or stock mixture to a
boil, cover tightly, reduce the heat, and simmer for
about 25 minutes, or until the celery is tender.
4 Heat the broiler to moderate. Drain the celery
and transfer to a heatproof serving dish.
5 Top with the remaining oil or butter, Parmesan,
almonds, and pepper. Broil until the almonds turn
golden, 1–2 minutes, and serve at once.

NUTRITIONAL INFORMATION

Amount per serving

Calories/(k/cal)	264/1104
Total fat (g)	22
% of calories	75
Sat. fat (g)	5
% of calories	15
Cholesterol (mg)	15
Total carb. (g)	4
Starch (g)	1
Fiber (g)	5
Protein (g)	13
Sodium (mg)	347

Rich source of calcium, magnesium,
phosphorus, potassium, vitamin E

HEALTH LINKS

Gout and rheumatoid arthritis,
pp. 80–81; Circulation and heart
health, pp. 82–5; Fluid retention,
p. 84

VARIATIONS

◆ *Cauliflower Amandine:
Use 1¼ lb (600g) cauliflower,
cut in quarters. Cook for
13 minutes.*
◆ *Spinach Amandine: Use
3¼ lb (1.5kg) fresh spinach.
Wash thoroughly and cook for
3–5 minutes in the water left
on the leaves after washing.*

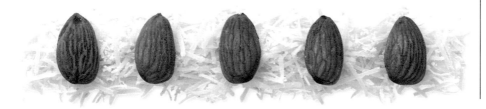

❖ Broccoli Stir-Fry ❖

Ingredients

2 tbsp light or dark soy sauce

2 tsp cornstarch or potato starch

2 tsp sugar or honey

1 tbsp apple juice or sherry

1 tbsp rice vinegar

2 tsp canola oil

6 shallots or 1 onion, thinly sliced

2 garlic cloves, thinly sliced

1½ inch (3.5cm) piece fresh
ginger, very thinly sliced

2 carrots, cut into matchsticks

1lb (450g) broccoli florets

1lb (450g) finely chopped mixed
vegetables, such as fava beans,
fennel, asparagus, bok choi or
napa, or whole bean sprouts

¼ cup (100g) unblanched
almonds and sunflower seeds

2 tsp sesame oil

*Bright green and orange vegetables are appetizing
and reflect a wide range of nutrients. Avoid preparing
the ingredients too far in advance or overcooking.*

1 Combine the soy sauce, cornstarch, sugar, juice, and
vinegar in a measuring cup and mix until smooth. Add
enough water to make 1 cup (250ml), stir, and set aside.
2 In a large skillet or wok, heat the canola oil until
sizzling hot. Add the shallots and garlic and stir-fry for
3–4 minutes.
3 Add the ginger, carrots, and broccoli. Then add
the mixed vegetables, ensuring that leafy vegetables,
such as bok choi, napa, or bean sprouts, are added last.
Stir-fry for 4–5 minutes. If the mixture looks too dry,
cover and reduce the heat for 1–2 minutes.
4 Add the almonds, sunflower seeds, and sesame oil
and stir-fry for 30 seconds.
5 Pour over the sauce, stirring steadily until the mixture
is boiling. Cook for another minute and serve at once.

Nutritional Information

Amount per serving

Calories/(k/cals)	339/1413
Total fat (g)	20
% of calories	53
Sat. fat (g)	2
% of calories	5
Cholesterol (mg)	0
Total carb. (g)	25
Starch (g)	10
Fiber (g)	10
Protein (g)	17
Sodium (mg)	462

*Rich source of carotenes, copper, folic
acid, iron, magnesium, phosphorus,
vitamins A, C, and E, zinc*

Health Links

Circulation and heart health, pp. 82–5
The body's defenses, p. 89

Variation

◆ *Broccoli & Tofu Stir-Fry:*
*Replace the almonds and
sunflower seeds with ½ lb
(200g) firm tofu, cut into cubes.*

❖ ODEN-STYLE STUFFED CABBAGE ❖

INGREDIENTS

½ cup (20g) dried shiitake mushrooms

12 large green cabbage leaves

½ lb (200g) firm, plain tofu or cooked kasha

½ lb (250g) ground pork

¼ lb (150g) scallions, finely sliced

1 tsp sesame oil

2 tbsp mirin, or sake plus 1 tsp sugar

¼ tsp sea salt

1 tsp sugar

12 long strips of leek, optional

1 large carrot, sliced

2¼ cups (500ml) vegetable stock, including the mushroom soaking water

1 tbsp light soy sauce

4 small hard-boiled eggs, optional

horseradish sauce and sweet rice vinegar, to serve

Oden is a light, Japanese style of vegetable cookery. This recipe provides the benefits of tofu and cabbage.

1 Place the dried mushrooms in a heatproof bowl and cover with 1¼ cups (300ml) boiling water. Let stand for 20–30 minutes.
2 Bring a large pan of water to a boil. Dip the cabbage leaves in for about 10 seconds until pliable. Drain and set aside.
3 Drain the mushrooms, reserving the soaking water, and slice very thin. Cut the tofu into 24 thin slices.
4 In a bowl, combine the mushrooms, pork, scallions, sesame oil, mirin, salt, and half of the sugar.
5 Lay each cabbage leaf flat, spread with some of the pork mixture, followed by 2 slices of tofu or 1 heaping tablespoon kasha. Fold the stem end over, tuck in the sides, and roll up. Secure with a leek strip, if using.
6 Place the carrot slices in a wide saucepan. Wedge the cabbage rolls together on top of the carrot slices.
7 In a saucepan, heat the stock, soy sauce, and the remaining sugar until nearly boiling. Pour over the rolls, cover, and cook for 15 minutes over moderate heat, turning once halfway through the cooking time.
8 Using a slotted spoon, place the cabbage rolls on a warmed serving dish. Pour over the cooking broth.
9 Garnish with the carrot slices and eggs, if using. Serve with horseradish sauce and sweet rice vinegar.

NUTRITIONAL INFORMATION

Amount per serving

Calories (kcal)	308
Total fat (g)	15
% of calories	44
Sat. fat (g)	4
% of calories	11
Cholesterol (mg)	237
Total carb. (g)	17
Starch (g)	1
Fiber (g)	5
Protein (g)	27
Sodium (mg)	542

Rich source of calcium, carotenes, folic acid, niacin, phosphorus, vitamins A, B₁₂, and C, zinc

HEALTH LINKS

Menopause, p. 87
The body's defenses, p. 89

VARIATIONS

◆ *Replace the pork with ½ lb (250g) fried or flavored tofu.*
◆ *Replace the vegetable stock with a Japanese seaweed-and-bonito fish stock, or* dashi, *see* Suimono Soup *recipe, p. 101.*

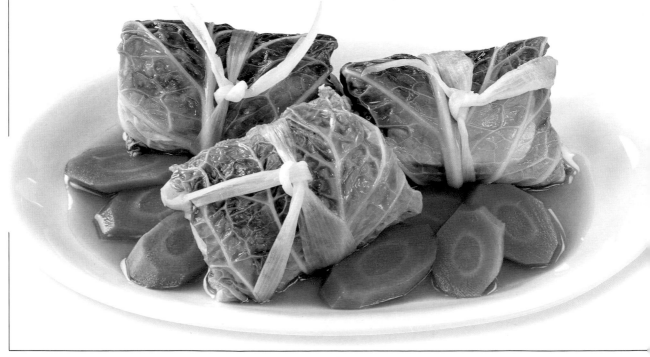

❖ NUT & CHERRY PILAF ❖

INGREDIENTS

2 tbsp sunflower oil
1 onion, thinly sliced
1 tbsp butter
pinch of saffron or turmeric, optional
2 cups (350g) long-grain rice, preferably brown basmati
¼ cup (40g) unblanched almonds
3 tbsp pine nuts or sunflower or pumpkin seeds
3 celery stalks, finely sliced
½ lb (250g) fresh or frozen cherries, pitted
1½ tsp ground cinnamon
1 tbsp lemon juice
½ cup (60g) chopped scallions
2 tbsp chopped fresh dill or mint
freshly ground black pepper
sea salt

Central Asia has hundreds of recipes for pilafs, which are colorful, aromatic rice dishes. They blend long-grain rice or bulgur wheat with different fruits, herbs, or nuts and sometimes meat.

1 In a heavy-bottomed saucepan, heat the oil, add the onion, and cook gently for 10 minutes, uncovered.
2 Add the butter, saffron or turmeric, if using, either ordinary long-grain or basmati rice, whole unblanched almonds, and pine nuts or sunflower or pumpkin seeds to the onion and stir for 2–3 minutes.
3 Add the celery, cherries, and cinnamon. Add double the volume of water for ordinary long-grain rice or 3¾ cups (850ml) water for basmati rice. Bring to a boil. Stir once, cover, reduce the heat to the lowest setting, and simmer for 20–45 minutes, or until all the water is absorbed.
4 When the rice is cooked, stir in the lemon juice, scallions, and fresh herbs. Season to taste and serve.

NUTRITIONAL INFORMATION

Amount per serving

Calories (kcal)	609
Total fat (g)	27
% of calories	39
Sat. fat (g)	5
% of calories	7
Cholesterol (mg)	9
Total carb. (g)	87
Starch (g)	7
Fiber (g)	3
Protein (g)	12
Sodium (mg)	56

Rich source of copper, phosphorus, vitamin E

HEALTH LINKS

Gout, p. 81; Heart health, pp. 82–5; Diabetic health, pp. 90–91

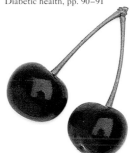

❖ FALAFEL ❖

INGREDIENTS

1½ cups (350g) chickpeas or white lima beans, dry weight
1 onion, finely chopped
6-8 scallions, finely chopped
1 large or 2 small garlic cloves, crushed
1 tsp ground cumin
2 tsp ground coriander seeds
freshly ground black pepper
½ tsp baking powder
½ tsp ground cayenne
1 egg, optional
4 tbsp extra-virgin olive oil

A lower fat version of this classic Middle Eastern dish, this recipe is made without deep frying. Serve with Low-Fat Hummus, see p. 140, and pita bread.

1 Soak the chickpeas or lima beans overnight.
2 Drain, rinse, and cover with fresh water. Bring to a boil, reduce the heat, simmer for 30 minutes, and drain.
3 In a food processor, grind the cooked beans into a fine paste with the onion, scallions, garlic, cumin, coriander seeds, pepper, baking powder, and cayenne. Add the egg if the mixture looks dry, to make it easier to form the mixture into balls.
4 Preheat the oven to 425°F/220°C. Heat half of the oil in a shallow baking dish.
5 Meanwhile, roll small amounts of the falafel mixture between your hands to form walnut-sized balls, then flatten each ball slightly. Heat the remaining oil in a thick-bottomed skillet and fry the falafel over high heat, turning often, to seal all the sides.
6 Wearing ovenmitts, transfer the falafel to the baking dish. Oven-fry for 10–15 minutes, shaking the dish often, until browned on all sides. Drain on paper towels and serve.

NUTRITIONAL INFORMATION

Amount per serving

Calories (kcal)	431
Total fat (g)	21
% of calories	43
Sat. fat (g)	3
% of calories	5
Cholesterol (mg)	0
Total carb. (g)	47
Starch (g)	39
Fiber (g)	10
Protein (g)	20
Sodium (mg)	98

Rich source of copper, folic acid, iron, magnesium, phosphorus, zinc

HEALTH LINKS

Heart health, pp. 82–5; Anemia, p. 85; Diabetic health, pp. 90–91

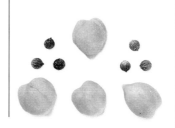

SIDE DISHES

WHEN COMPARED TO plain-cooked vegetables, side dishes that can transform vegetables and legumes into something special are a useful way to gain new enthusiasts, even among those who do not like their "greens." In this recipe selection the emphasis is on the colorful – with ingredients such as red cabbage, split red lentils, tomatoes, orange-fleshed sweet potatoes, and winter squash – and mellow-tasting, slowly cooked dishes, for example, roast onions. The vegetable side dishes are ideal to serve as an additional side dish, and a good way to encourage eating an extra serving of vegetables with their protective properties. Unlike green vegetables, most can be cooked in advance and reheated successfully. Side dishes made with legumes give substance to a light meal such as a salad. They also provide iron and protein, and perfectly balance a vegetable main course. Dried legumes are underused because most need presoaking, but they are easy to cook, highly versatile, tastier, and more nutritious and economical than canned versions.

LIMA BEANS WITH SAGE & GARLIC

Comforting and aromatic, lima beans gently simmered with garlic complement a vegetable main course.

Sage and garlic are both herbal antiseptics and give a savory "meatiness" to delicately flavored lima beans

Lima beans are a good source of soluble fiber, B vitamins, potassium, and iron

❖ Lima Beans with Sage & Garlic ❖

Ingredients

1½ cups (250g) lima beans, dry weight

2–3 tbsp extra-virgin olive oil

2 bay leaves

2½ cups (600ml) water

1 garlic clove, finely sliced

4 sage leaves, roughly chopped

juice of ½ lemon

freshly ground black pepper

sea salt

2–3 tbsp chopped fresh herbs, such as chives or parsley, to garnish

Using a good quality extra-virgin olive oil is the key to success in this Greek-style recipe.

1 Soak the lima beans overnight, then drain.

2 In a large saucepan, heat 1 tablespoon of the olive oil, add the lima beans, and cook over low heat, stirring occasionally, for 10 minutes.

3 Add the bay leaves and water and bring to a boil. Reduce the heat and simmer gently, covered, for about 40 minutes, or until the beans are tender. Drain, reserving the cooking liquid.

4 In the same pan, heat the remaining oil, add the garlic and sage, rubbing the leaves between your fingers to release their flavor. Cook over medium heat until sizzling. Stir in the beans and cook, covered, over low heat for a few minutes. As they become dry, add a few spoonfuls of the cooking liquid.

5 Add the lemon juice and season to taste. Garnish with the chopped herbs and serve warm, not hot.

Nutritional Information

Amount per serving

Calories (kcal)	268
Total fat (g)	10
% of calories	35
Sat. fat (g)	2
% of calories	5
Cholesterol (mg)	0
Total carb. (g)	33
Starch (g)	29
Fiber (g)	10
Protein (g)	12
Sodium (mg)	26

Rich source of copper, iron, magnesium, phosphorus, potassium, zinc

Health Links

Heart health, pp. 82–5
Diabetic health, pp. 90–91

❖ Spiced Winter Squash ❖

Ingredients

2¼ lb (1kg) winter squash or pumpkin

1½ tbsp extra-virgin olive or sesame oil or 1 tbsp butter

1 large onion, finely chopped

3 tsp grated fresh ginger

1 cup (250ml) water

¼ tsp ground cinnamon

freshly ground black pepper

sea salt

Squash, onion, ginger, and cinnamon are perfect flavor partners and make a colorful dish that is rich in carotenes.

1 Preheat the oven to 375°F/190°C.

2 Halve the squash or pumpkin, place it cut side down in a lightly greased shallow baking dish. Bake for 30–45 minutes, or until the flesh is tender.

3 Meanwhile, in a large saucepan, heat the oil or butter and gently cook the onion over the lowest heat setting until golden and translucent, at least 25 minutes. Add the ginger, stir for 1–2 minutes, remove from the heat, and set aside.

4 Scoop the seeds out of the center of the cooked squash or pumpkin. Using a large spoon, scoop out the flesh and stir it into the onion and ginger mixture.

5 Add the water to the pan, bring to a boil and cover. Reduce the heat and simmer for 20 minutes, stirring occasionally. Add a little water if the mixture is too dry.

6 Process or blend all into a smooth purée, or process only part of the mixture if you prefer a coarser version. Add the cinnamon, season to taste, and serve.

Nutritional Information

Amount per serving

Calories (kcal)	150
Total fat (g)	4
% of calories	25
Sat. fat (g)	0.6
% of calories	4
Cholesterol (mg)	0
Total carb. (g)	26
Starch (g)	20
Fiber (g)	6
Protein (g)	3
Sodium (mg)	9

Rich source of carotenes, magnesium, potassium, vitamin C

Health Link

Circulation and heart health, pp. 82–5

❖ BRAISED RED CABBAGE ❖

INGREDIENTS

1 red cabbage, finely shredded
1 tbsp sunflower oil
2 onions, finely chopped
2 large cooking apples, peeled and roughly chopped
juice of 1–2 lemons
3 cloves
5 black or white peppercorns
2 tsp honey
sea salt

Colorful sweet-and-sour braised red cabbage can attract new enthusiasts to cabbage.

1 Place the cabbage in a heatproof bowl and pour over boiling water to cover. Let stand for 1 minute and drain.
2 Heat the oil in a large saucepan, add the onions, and cook very gently, uncovered, for 10 minutes.
3 Add the cabbage, apples, juice of 1 lemon, cloves, peppercorns, and honey. Stir, bring to a boil, cover tightly, and reduce the heat to the lowest setting. Simmer for about 1¼ hours, stirring occasionally.
4 Remove the cloves and peppercorns. Check the flavoring, adding more lemon juice or honey, if desired. Season to taste and serve.

NUTRITIONAL INFORMATION

Amount per serving

Calories (kcal)	13
Total fat (g)	
% of calories	2
Sat. fat (g)	
% of calories	
Cholesterol (mg)	
Total carb. (g)	2
Starch (g)	trac
Fiber (g)	
Protein (g)	
Sodium (mg)	1

Rich source of folic acid, vitamin C

HEALTH LINK

The body's defenses, p. 89

❖ ROAST ONIONS ❖

INGREDIENTS

4 large onions, each weighing about ½ lb (200g)
2 tsp sunflower oil
1¼ cups (300ml) water or stock, or half wine and water/stock
¼ lb (120g) low-fat soft cheese, to serve, optional

Let onions be the star of a recipe for once. In this elegant, simple dish, onions are gently baked until they become mild and melting.

1 Preheat the oven to 350°F/180°C.
2 Remove any roots from the base of the onions but do not peel them. Place the onions in a baking dish and brush them with oil.
3 Pour the water, stock, or wine around the onions. Bake for 1½–2 hours, basting with the juices occasionally, until tender.
4 Cut a deep cross in the top of each onion and peel back the outer layers. Place a dollop of soft cheese, if using, in the top of each onion, and serve.

NUTRITIONAL INFORMATION

Amount per serving

Calories (kcal)	9
Total fat (g)	3
% of calories	2
Sat. fat (g)	
% of calories	
Cholesterol (mg)	
Total carb. (g)	1
Starch (g)	
Fiber (g)	3
Protein (g)	
Sodium (mg)	

HEALTH LINKS

Respiratory infections, p. 76
Circulation and heart health, pp. 82–5
Diabetic health, pp. 90–91

❖ SWEET POTATO CHIPS ❖

INGREDIENTS

1¼ lb (600g) orange-fleshed sweet potatoes
1–2 tbsp canola oil

This is a delicious way to bring colorful sweet potatoes into everyday use, gaining the benefit of their exceptional vitamin E and carotenes content.

1 Peel the sweet potatoes and then cut into fat chips about ½ inch (1cm) square.
2 In a large, heavy-bottomed skillet, heat the oil and stir-fry the potatoes over high heat for 8–9 minutes, until just tender and blistered in places.

NUTRITIONAL INFORMATION

Amount per serving

Calories (kcal)	175
Total fat (g)	5
% of calories	28
Sat. fat (g)	1
% of calories	2
Cholesterol (mg)	0
Total carb. (g)	32
Starch (g)	23
Fiber (g)	4
Protein (g)	2
Sodium (mg)	60

Rich source of carotenes, potassium, vitamins A, C, and E

HEALTH LINK

Heart health, pp. 82–5

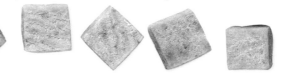

❖ DHAL ❖

1 cup (250g) split red lentils, rinsed

½ tsp ground turmeric

1¼ cups (600ml) water

1 tbsp extra-virgin olive oil

1 onion, finely chopped

1 green chili pepper, seeded and finely chopped

1 small fresh tomato, chopped

1½ inch (3cm) piece fresh ginger, sliced very thin

2 garlic cloves, crushed

1 tsp cumin seeds, crushed

seeds of 3 cardamom pods, crushed

3–4 tbsp chopped fresh cilantro, to garnish

Dhal is a classic but not fiery hot Indian dish, and is an easy way to enjoy lentils, one of the most nutritious of legumes, high in iron, thiamin, and zinc.

1 In a large saucepan, bring the lentils, turmeric, and water to a boil, cover, reduce the heat, and cook gently for 20–25 minutes, until tender.

2 Meanwhile, in another saucepan, heat half of the oil and add the onion. Cook over low heat, stirring often, for about 10 minutes, until golden. Add the chili pepper and tomatoes and cook over medium heat, stirring often, for about 10 minutes, until a paste forms.

3 In a small skillet, heat the remaining oil and add the ginger, garlic, cumin, and cardamom. Cook for 2 minutes.

4 Stir the onion mixture, the spices, and half the cilantro into the lentils.

5 Check the seasoning, garnish with the remaining chopped cilantro and serve.

NUTRITIONAL INFORMATION

Amount per serving

Calories (kcal)	259
Total fat (g)	5
% of calories	18
Sat. fat (g)	1
% of calories	3
Cholesterol (mg)	0
Total carb. (g)	40
Starch (g)	33
Fiber (g)	4
Protein (g)	16
Sodium (mg)	34

Rich source of copper, iron, phosphorus, thiamin, zinc

HEALTH LINKS

Respiratory infections, p. 76
Circulation and heart health, pp. 82–5
Anemia, p. 85
Diabetic health, pp. 90–91

❖ BAKED TOMATOES ❖

4 small beefsteak or 8 garden tomatoes

1 garlic clove, crushed

freshly ground black pepper

large pinch of sea salt

3 tbsp finely chopped fresh basil, chives, or parsley

2 tsp extra-virgin olive oil

An easy, Italian-style recipe that intensifies the flavor of tomatoes and retains their high antioxidant content.

1 Preheat the oven to 425°F/225°C. Oil a shallow baking dish.

2 Turn the tomatoes upside down and slice across each tomato, about ½ inch (1cm) down from the base, to make a "lid." Set the lids aside and place the tomatoes in the baking dish cut side up.

3 Using a sharp knife, make several cuts across the surface of each tomato. Spread the tops with the garlic, pepper, salt, herbs, and 1 teaspoon of the oil.

4 Put the lids back on and dribble the rest of the oil over the tomatoes. Bake on the top shelf for 20–25 minutes, or until the tomatoes are soft but not collapsing, and starting to blister on top. Serve them warm, not straight from the oven.

NUTRITIONAL INFORMATION

Amount per serving

Calories (kcal)	98
Total fat (g)	8
% of calories	74
Sat. fat (g)	1
% of calories	11
Cholesterol (mg)	0
Total carb. (g)	5
Starch (g)	trace
Fiber (g)	2
Protein (g)	1
Sodium (mg)	112

Rich source of carotenes, vitamin C

HEALTH LINK

The body's defenses, p. 89

DESSERTS

THINK OF A HEALTHY dessert and you probably picture fresh fruit. But think of your favorite dessert and you probably imagine something more "wicked." The desserts that are featured here bridge the gap: they are alluring but still surprisingly low in sugar and fat. The selection is also highly flexible, using techniques that work with a variety of ingredients. These recipes prove that you do not need high-fat cream or pastry to make a special dessert. Dessert is a perfect time to eat more fruit, with its important health bonuses. We think of fruit as mainly providing vitamin C, but it is also an outstanding source of soluble fiber, potassium, beta-carotene, and other nutrients. The key to keeping sugar content low is to mix a tart fruit with another that is naturally very sweet, for example, cranberries with pears. Dried apricots are especially useful. To retain maximum nutrient value, minimize cooking times and make use of the cooking liquid.

SUMMER PUDDING
This handsome pudding is almost fat-free, with the health benefits of berries.

Cherries can help some gout sufferers

Purple berries derive their color from anthocyanins, which have antioxidant properties

❖ SUMMER PUDDING ❖

INGREDIENTS

6 slices whole-wheat bread, crusts removed

1lb 10oz (750g) mixed fruits, such as 1lb 2oz (500g) fresh or frozen berries, for example, black currants, bilberries, blueberries, cranberries, or pitted cherries and 9oz (250g) sweet fruits, for example, apricots and nectarines, pitted and roughly chopped

1–2 tbsp honey to taste

sprig of mint or fruit slices, to decorate

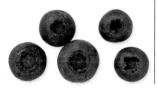

This molded pudding creates a sense of occasion, but it is among the easiest desserts to make, and the lowest in fat. Every ingredient has a health bonus.

1 Line a 4½ cup (1 liter) pudding mold or soufflé dish with the bread slices, trimming them as necessary to fit the bottom and sides. Reserve 1–2 slices for the top.
2 Put the washed fruit in a saucepan with 1 cup (250ml) water. Bring to a boil, reduce the heat, and simmer for about 5 minutes, until soft but not mushy. Cool a little and add honey to taste.
3 Reserve 3 tablespoons of the juice from the cooked fruit. Pour the remainder of the juice and cooked fruit into the pudding mold. Top with the remaining bread.
4 Place a saucer over the pudding mold (it should neatly fit inside the rim) and place a 1lb weight on top. Chill for at least 5 hours before serving.
5 Invert the pudding onto a plate. If any patches of bread have not been colored by the fruit, use a pastry brush to coat with the reserved juice. Decorate with a sprig of mint or a slice of fruit and serve.

NUTRITIONAL INFORMATION

Amount per serving	
Calories (kcal)	140
Total fat (g)	1
% of calories	5
Sat. fat (g)	1
% of calories	1
Cholesterol (mg)	0
Total carb. (g)	31
Starch (g)	12
Fiber (g)	7
Protein (g)	1
Sodium (mg)	177

Rich source of copper, vitamin C

HEALTH LINKS

Eye health, p. 77; Constipation, p. 78; Gout, pp. 81; Circulation and heart health, pp. 82–5

VARIATION

❖ *Winter pudding: use 1lb 2oz (500g) apples and pears, cored and chopped, and 9oz (250g) fresh or frozen cranberries.*

❖ BAKED GINGER BANANAS ❖

INGREDIENTS

2 tbsp golden raisins, optional

2 tsp butter

4 large firm bananas, halved lengthwise

2 pieces preserved stem ginger, thinly sliced

1 tbsp syrup from preserved stem ginger

2 tbsp orange juice

2 tbsp rum

12–15 strands orange zest

VARIATIONS

❖ *Replace the bananas with other fruits, such as halved peaches, apricots, nectarines, apples, or pears, and bake in the same way.*
❖ *Add 1–2 tsp ground cinnamon.*
❖ *Replace the rum with 4 tbsp orange juice and 1 tsp honey.*

This quick dessert offers a classic blend of flavors and shows that you can enjoy the taste of butter, while using only a small quantity.

1 Preheat the oven to 400°F/200°C. If using the golden raisins, place them in a cup and cover with boiling water. Let soak for 5 minutes and drain.
2 Meanwhile, put the butter in a shallow baking dish just wide enough to hold the bananas in a single layer, and place in the oven until the butter has melted. Remove, add the banana halves, and brush with the melted butter. Sprinkle the bananas with the raisins, if using, ginger, syrup, orange juice, rum, and orange zest.
3 Bake for 15 minutes, basting 2–3 times. Serve hot.
4 If you want to flambé the bananas, bake with only 1 tablespoon rum. Before serving, warm the remaining rum by holding it in a metal ladle over a low flame. Pour over the bananas and light it with a match.

NUTRITIONAL INFORMATION

Amount per serving	
Calories (kcal)	169
Total fat (g)	2
% of calories	13
Sat. fat (g)	1
% of calories	8
Cholesterol (mg)	6
Total carb. (g)	33
Starch (g)	3
Fiber (g)	1
Protein (g)	2
Sodium (mg)	31

HEALTH LINKS

Diarrhea, pp. 78–9; Nausea, pp. 78–9; Circulation, pp. 82–5

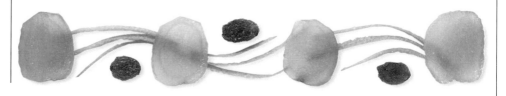

❖ PINEAPPLE FONDUE ❖

Eating chocolate in moderation is not unhealthy. In this recipe, the cool pineapple chunks harden the chocolate sauce.

INGREDIENTS

1 small pineapple

3½ oz (100g) good-quality semisweet chocolate, broken into squares

2 tbsp light cream

2 tsp rum or brandy, optional

2–3 tbsp low-fat milk

1 Peel and cut the pineapple into neat, bite-sized chunks and chill, wrapped, while you make the chocolate sauce.
2 Fit a small heatproof bowl on top of a saucepan of simmering water. Add all the remaining ingredients except for 1 tablespoon milk to the bowl.
3 As the mixture heats very gently, stir it constantly, until you have a smooth chocolate sauce. Add the remaining milk if needed to give the mixture a thick liquid consistency. Do not overheat.
4 Divide the sauce among 4 small, warmed cups.
5 Place a small cup of chocolate sauce on each dish with a share of pineapple chunks and a fork to dip the pineapple chunks into the sauce, and serve.

NUTRITIONAL INFORMATION

Amount per serving

Calories (kcal)	22
Total fat (g)	
% of calories	3
Sat. fat (g)	
% of calories	2
Cholesterol (mg)	
Total carb. (g)	3
Starch (g)	
Fiber (g)	
Protein (g)	
Sodium (mg)	1

Rich source of copper, vitamin C

HEALTH LINKS

Digestion, pp. 78–9
Wound-healing, p. 88

VARIATION

◆ *Use 1lb 5oz (600g) unpitted fresh cherries.*

❖ APRICOT ALMOND FOOL ❖

Dried apricots, yogurt, and almonds make an easy dessert with a high nutritional value. The first boiling of the apricots helps remove most preservative.

INGREDIENTS

1 cup (250g) dried apricots

2¼ cups (500ml) low-fat plain yogurt with active cultures

1 tbsp honey, optional

¼ cup (40g) unblanched almonds, roughly chopped or sliced

fresh mint or edible flowers, to decorate, optional

VARIATIONS

◆ *Apple Almond Fool: Replace the apricots with 1½ lb (700g) cored and roughly chopped apples and a seedless lemon slice. In a large saucepan, bring 1¼ cups (300ml) water to a boil and add the apples. Cover, reduce the heat, and simmer for 6–12 minutes, or until just tender. Discard the lemon and continue with the recipe from step 3.*
◆ *Purée the fruit with 2 pieces preserved stem ginger.*

1 Place the apricots in a saucepan, cover with cold water, bring to a boil, and simmer for 5 minutes. Drain and add fresh cold water to cover the apricots.
2 Return to a boil, cover, reduce the heat, and simmer for 20 minutes, or until the apricots are soft.
3 Cool slightly. Process or blend with just enough of the cooking water to make a thick purée. Cool until lukewarm.
4 Stir in the yogurt and honey, if using. Chill until ready to serve.
5 Just before serving, heat the almonds in an ungreased skillet over low heat for 2–3 minutes, until just starting to turn golden. Sprinkle the hot almonds over the fool, decorate with the fresh mint or edible flowers, if using, and serve.

NUTRITIONAL INFORMATION

Amount per serving

Calories (kcal)	320
Total fat (g)	7
% of calories	27
Sat. fat (g)	1
% of calories	4
Cholesterol (mg)	5
Total carb. (g)	33
Starch (g)	trace
Fiber (g)	5
Protein (g)	11
Sodium (mg)	114

Rich source of calcium, copper, phosphorus, potassium, vitamin E

HEALTH LINKS

Constipation, p. 78
Gastroenteritis, p. 79
Heart health, pp. 82–5
Yeast infections, p. 87

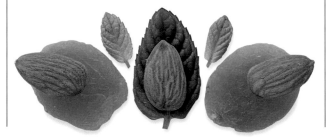

❖ REAL MUESLI ❖

INGREDIENTS

3 tbsp old-fashioned oatmeal, preferably, or 4 tbsp rolled oats

¼ cup (180ml) low-fat plain yogurt with active cultures

4 tsp lemon juice

4 tbsp honey

1lb 12oz (800g) red-skinned apples, well scrubbed

4 tbsp finely chopped unblanched almonds or hazelnuts

The original muesli recipe from the Swiss naturopath Dr. Bircher-Benner is an apple dish, not a breakfast cereal, and makes a tasty dessert.

1 Soak the oatmeal or rolled oats overnight in ½ cup (135ml) water.
2 In a bowl, mix the yogurt with the lemon juice, and stir in the soaked oatmeal or rolled oats and the honey.
3 Coarsely grate the unpeeled apple into the mixture, stirring often to prevent discoloration.
4 Sprinkle with the nuts and serve.

NUTRITIONAL INFORMATION

Amount per serving

Calories (kcal)	273
Total fat (g)	10
% of calories	32
Sat. fat (g)	1
% of calories	3
Cholesterol (mg)	2
Total carb. (g)	42
Starch (g)	5
Fiber (g)	5
Protein (g)	7
Sodium (mg)	48

Rich source of phosphorus, vitamin E

HEALTH LINKS

Constipation, p. 78; Diarrhea, pp. 78–9; Peptic ulcers, p. 79; Heart health, pp. 82–5; Yeast infections, p. 87; Diabetic health, pp. 90–91

❖ HONEY & LEMON CHEESECAKE ❖

INGREDIENTS

For the base

1 cup (50g) fresh whole wheat bread crumbs

¼ cup (25g) rolled oats

2 tbsp (25g) soft margarine or softened butter

3 tbsp freshly ground unblanched almonds or a mixture of almonds and sunflower seeds, plus 1–3 drops almond extract

For the filling

1lb 2oz (500g) medium or low-fat smooth soft cheese

2 tbsp cold-pressed honey or honeycomb

½ cup–⅔ cup (100–150ml) thick, low-fat plain yogurt with active cultures

¼ cup (40g) raisins or dried apricots, chopped

4–5 drops vanilla extract

grated zest of 1 lemon

For the topping

½ lb (225g) mixed fresh fruit, such as pitted apricots, cherries, and blueberries

The simplicity of this creamy-textured cheesecake transforms this dessert from a special-occasion dish into one that can be enjoyed anytime. High in protein, it is ideal to follow a salad.

1 Preheat the oven to 375°F/190°C. To make the cheesecake base, combine the bread crumbs and oats in a bowl. Fork in the margarine or butter until well mixed. Stir in the almonds and sunflower seeds, if using, into the bread-crumb mixture with the almond extract.
2 Place in a 7 inch (18cm) greased springform pan, pressing down with a fork until smooth. Bake for 20 minutes.
3 To make the filling, mix the soft cheese with the honey and enough yogurt to make a smooth, thick paste.
4 Stir in the dried fruit, vanilla extract, and lemon zest. Check that the mixture is sweet enough. Spread on top of the base and chill for at least 1 hour before serving.
5 Top with fresh fruit and serve.

NUTRITIONAL INFORMATION

Amount per serving

Calories (kcal)	445
Total fat (g)	28
% of calories	57
Sat. fat (g)	14
% of calories	27
Cholesterol (mg)	54
Total carb. (g)	33
Starch (g)	9
Fiber (g)	3
Protein (g)	17
Sodium (mg)	150

Rich source of phosphorus, vitamins A and E

HEALTH LINKS

Digestion, pp. 78–9
Skin health, p. 88
Urinary tract infections, p. 92

❖ CRANBERRY & APRICOT COMPOTE ❖

INGREDIENTS

1 cup (250g) dried apricots
2 cups (250g) fresh or frozen cranberries
1 tbsp honey, optional
zest from 1 lemon, to decorate

VARIATIONS

◆ *Replace the cranberries with 12–14oz (350–400g) black currants or pitted cherries.*
◆ *Replace the dried apricots with dried peaches or pears and stew with a seedless lemon slice.*

Dried apricots are a healthy way of sweetening cranberries, and the mix of color is luscious.

1 Place the apricots in a saucepan, cover with water, bring to a boil, and simmer for 5 minutes. Drain and add fresh cold water to cover the apricots.
2 Return to a boil, reduce the heat, and simmer, covered, for 20 minutes or until tender.
3 Add the cranberries, return to a boil, and continue cooking over medium heat for 6–8 minutes, until the cranberries have burst.
4 Pour into a serving dish with just enough of the cooking liquid to cover. Add honey to taste and decorate with the lemon zest.
5 Let stand for a few minutes to allow the flavors to blend together. Serve hot or cold.

NUTRITIONAL INFORMATION

Amount per serving

Calories (kcal)	108
Total fat (g)	1
% of calories	4
Sat. fat (g)	0
% of calories	0
Cholesterol (mg)	0
Total carb. (g)	30
Starch (g)	0
Fiber (g)	6
Protein (g)	3
Sodium (mg)	10

Rich source of potassium

HEALTH LINKS

Constipation, p. 78
Heart health, pp. 82–5
Urinary tract infections, p. 92

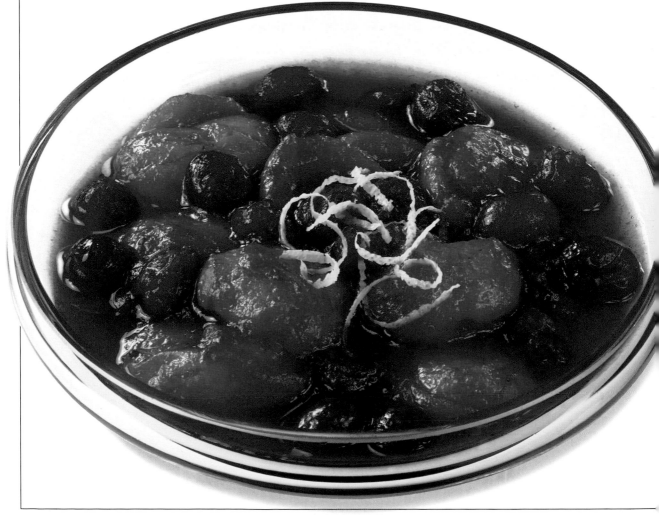

❖ KISSEL ❖

INGREDIENTS

1lb 2oz (500g) mixed fresh or frozen berries, such as black currants, bilberries, blueberries, or cranberries, and pitted cherries

9oz (250g) summer fruits, such as peaches, apricots, or nectarines, pitted and roughly chopped

⅔ cup (150ml) water

1–3 tbsp honey, to taste

2 tbsp arrowroot or cornstarch

This is a perfect summer dessert. Arrowroot gives a subtle shimmer to the berries, and mixing them with sweeter fruits reduces the need for added sugar.

1 In a large saucepan, bring the fruit to a boil with the water. Cover, reduce the heat, and simmer for about 5 minutes, or until the fruit is barely soft. The amount of liquid in the pan will increase.
2 Remove the mixture from the heat. Stir in the honey to taste; black currants and cranberries require more sweetening than most other berries.
3 Mix the arrowroot with a little water to make a smooth paste. Add to the fruit, stirring constantly.
4 Return to a boil, stirring, and simmer for 2–3 minutes, until the liquid thickens and becomes clear.
5 Pour into a serving dish and chill until lightly set, 1–2 hours. Serve within 24 hours.

NUTRITIONAL INFORMATION

Amount per serving	
Calories (kcal)	119
Total fat (g)	trace
% of calories	1
Sat. fat (g)	0
% of calories	0
Cholesterol (mg)	0
Total carb. (g)	29
Starch (g)	7
Fiber (g)	4
Protein (g)	2
Sodium (mg)	4

Rich source of vitamin C

HEALTH LINKS

Eye health, p. 77
Circulation and heart health, pp. 82–5
Urinary tract infections, p. 92

❖ SUNFLOWER, APPLE & APRICOT CRUMBLE ❖

INGREDIENTS

For the filling

¼ cup (50g) dried apricots

1lb 2oz (500g) fresh fruit, such as apples, cherries, and apricots, pitted and roughly chopped and used individually or mixed

For the topping

⅓ cup (50g) whole-wheat flour

1½ tbsp soft margarine

1 tbsp skim milk powder

¼ cup (25g) sunflower seeds, coarsely ground

¼ cup (25g) rolled oats

4 tsp brown sugar or fruit sugar

A classic crumble, with less fat and sugar than traditional recipes, this is an excellent way to encourage the eating of more fruit all year.

1 Preheat the oven to 375°F/190°C.
2 Place the apricots in a saucepan, cover with water, bring to a boil, and simmer for 5 minutes. Drain and add fresh cold water to cover the apricots.
3 Return to a boil, reduce the heat, and simmer, covered, for 20 minutes, until tender.
4 Add the remaining fruit to the apricots and cook, covered, for 5 minutes.
5 Drain the fruit, reserving the liquid. Cut each of the dried apricots into 3–4 pieces. Place the fruit in a baking dish with ⅔ cup (150ml) of the cooking liquid.
6 To make the topping, put the flour in a bowl and cut in the margarine. Stir in the milk powder, sunflower seeds, oats, and all but 1 teaspoon of the sugar.
7 Spread the topping over the fruit and sprinkle with the remaining sugar. Bake for 15 minutes, or until golden, and serve.

NUTRITIONAL INFORMATION

Amount per serving	
Calories (kcal)	250
Total fat (g)	9
% of calories	31
Sat. fat (g)	2
% of calories	7
Cholesterol (mg)	1
Total carb. (g)	39
Starch (g)	13
Fiber (g)	4
Protein (g)	6
Sodium (mg)	70

Rich source of vitamin E

HEALTH LINKS

Constipation, p. 78
Heart health, pp. 82–5

VARIATION

◆ *Use 1lb 2oz (500g) black currants or cranberries, mixed with ½ cup (100g) stewed dried apricots and honey to taste.*

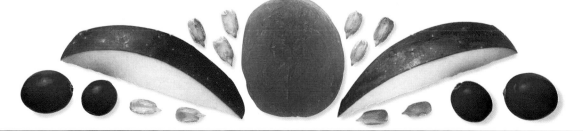

QUICK BREADS & CAKES

ONE OF THE JOYS of healthier eating is that you are urged to eat more starchy foods, which can include cakes and muffins when you use recipes like these. Unlike many cake recipes, which need a high proportion of fat or sugar to achieve texture or flavor, in these recipes fat and added sugar are minimized, and they work very well with whole-wheat flour. That does not mean they taste peculiar or are difficult to make: the huge heritage of baking has always had some recipes like these, buried among those for pound cakes and pastries. Generous amounts of fruits and spices give moist, rich flavors to baking recipes, and citrus fruits are valuable for adding a fresh tang. For cakes requiring whole-wheat flour, fineground is best. Flours vary in how much liquid they absorb. Unless otherwise stated, add liquid until you obtain a "dropping consistency," meaning that the mixture drops, rather than flows, off of the mixing spoon.

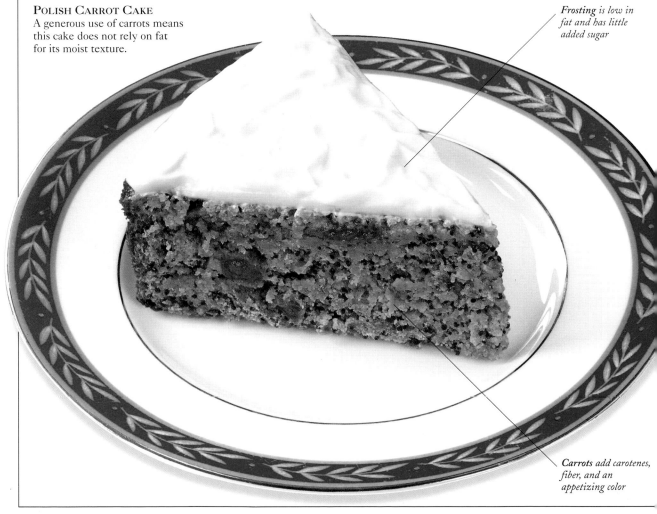

POLISH CARROT CAKE
A generous use of carrots means this cake does not rely on fat for its moist texture.

Frosting is low in fat and has little added sugar

Carrots add carotenes, fiber, and an appetizing color

❖ POLISH CARROT CAKE ❖

INGREDIENTS

oil to coat the pan

For the cake

½ cup (115ml) clear honey
3 tbsp soft sunflower margarine
½ cup (75g) golden raisins
½ lb (250g) finely grated carrots
grated zest of 1 lemon
⅔ cup (140ml) low-fat plain yogurt with active cultures
2 eggs, beaten
1½ cups (170g) all-purpose whole-wheat flour with 1½ tsp baking powder
3 tbsp crushed poppy seeds
1 tsp ground cinnamon

For the frosting

¼ lb (125g) low-fat fromage frais or smooth soft cheese
2 tsp honey
2 drops vanilla extract

A large slice of this super-moist cake has food value similar to that of a main course. Makes 10 slices.

1 Preheat the oven to 350°F/180°C. Oil a 7 inch (18cm) square or an 8 inch (20cm) round cake pan.
2 In a large saucepan, gently heat the honey, margarine, and the golden raisins.
3 Remove from the heat, stir in the carrots, lemon zest, yogurt, and eggs.
4 Sift in the flour with the baking powder and mix well. Stir in the poppy seeds and cinnamon.
5 Transfer to the cake pan, bake for 1 hour, then reduce the temperature to 300°F/150°C and bake for 30 minutes, until the edges of the cake begin to come away from the sides of the pan.
6 Cool the cake in the pan for 20 minutes, then invert it onto a wire rack.
7 To make the frosting, mix the ingredients together in a bowl until completely blended. Using a spatula or knife, spread the frosting over the cake.
8 Serve the cake cut into thin slices. Store in a covered container in the refrigerator. Eat within 4 days.

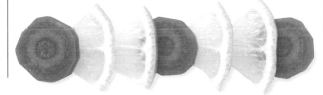

NUTRITIONAL INFORMATION

Amount per serving

Calories (kcal)	190
Total fat (g)	8
% of calories	34
Sat. fat (g)	2
% of calories	9
Cholesterol (mg)	40
Total carb. (g)	30
Starch (g)	11
Fiber (g)	2
Protein (g)	6
Sodium (mg)	139

Rich source of carotenes, phosphorus, vitamins A and B12

HEALTH LINKS

Constipation, p. 78
Heart health, pp. 82–5

❖ GINGERBREAD WITH ALMONDS ❖

INGREDIENTS

oil to coat the pan
½ cup (170g) molasses
3 tbsp sunflower margarine
1¼ cups (300ml) low-fat milk
2–4 pieces preserved stem ginger in syrup, chopped
½ cup (75g) golden raisins
1¾ cups (225g) whole-wheat flour
2 tsp baking powder
2 tsp ground ginger
1 tsp pie spice
⅓ cup (50g) medium oatmeal or oat bran
3 tbsp unblanched almonds, roughly chopped

This is an old-fashioned gingerbread, with a substantial level of ginger. For the best flavor, keep for 3–4 days before eating. Makes 15 slices.

1 Preheat the oven to 350°F/180°C. Lightly oil a 2lb (1kg) loaf pan.
2 In a large saucepan, gently heat the molasses and margarine, until liquid. Stir in the milk, ginger, and golden raisins. Remove from the heat.
3 In a mixing bowl, sift the flour with the baking powder, ground ginger, and mixed spice. Stir in the oatmeal or oat bran.
4 Stir the flour mixture into the molasses and ginger mixture. Mix quickly but thoroughly.
5 Pour the mixture into the prepared pan. Sprinkle with the almonds. Bake for 1 hour, or until a skewer inserted into the center comes out clean.
6 Let rest in the pan until just warm, then invert it onto a wire rack. Store in an airtight container.

NUTRITIONAL INFORMATION

Amount per serving

Calories (kcal)	153
Total fat (g)	5
% of calories	30
Sat. fat (g)	1
% of calories	7
Cholesterol (mg)	2
Total carb. (g)	25
Starch (g)	12
Fiber (g)	2
Protein (g)	4
Sodium (mg)	114

Rich source of phosphorus

HEALTH LINKS

Nausea, pp. 78–9
Circulation and heart health, pp. 82–5

❖ CRANBERRY FRUITCAKE ❖

INGREDIENTS

¼ cup (50g) dried apricots
½ cup (100g) prunes, pitted
scant 1 cup (200ml) water
oil to coat the pan
2 tbsp whiskey or orange juice
5 tbsp (75g) soft margarine or butter, or a mixture
2 tbsp honey
3 eggs, beaten
zest and juice of 1 lemon
1½ cups (225g) dark raisins, golden raisins, and currants
⅓ cup (75g) candied citrus peel
2 cups (250g) fresh cranberries
3 tbsp pumpkin seeds
1¼ cups (225g) whole-wheat flour
2 tsp baking powder
1½ tsp pie spice

Studded with brilliant red cranberries and green pumpkin seeds, this is a moist cake that is lower in fat than most fruitcakes. Makes 20 slices.

1 In a small saucepan, bring the apricots and prunes to a boil in the water. Cover, reduce the heat, and let them simmer for 15 minutes, or until soft.
2 Preheat the oven to 350°F/180°C. Lightly oil a 7 inch (18cm) square or an 8 inch (20cm) round cake pan.
3 In a food processor or blender, purée the fruit mixture until smooth, adding the whiskey or juice.
4 Transfer to a large mixing bowl. Add the margarine, honey, eggs, lemon zest and juice, raisins, currants, citrus peel, cranberries, and pumpkin seeds and mix together.
5 Sift in the flour, the baking powder, and mixed spice. Stir in the bran left in the sifter, except for 2 tablespoons. Mix well but quickly.
6 Spoon the mixture into the pan, smoothing the top. Bake on the center shelf of the oven for 30 minutes, then reduce the heat to 325°F/160°C for 1–1½ hours, or until a skewer inserted into the center comes out clean.
7 Cool the cake in the pan for 10 minutes, then invert it onto a wire rack. Cut into slices and serve. Store in a cool place and eat within 3 weeks.

NUTRITIONAL INFORMATION

Amount per serving

Calories (kcal)	150
Total fat (g)	6
% of calories	34
Sat. fat (g)	1
% of calories	8
Cholesterol (mg)	29
Total carb. (g)	22
Starch (g)	8
Fiber (g)	2
Protein (g)	3
Sodium (mg)	91

Rich source of phosphorus

HEALTH LINKS

Constipation, p. 78
Heart health, pp. 82–5

VARIATIONS

◆ Decorate the cake with patterns of mixed fruit and nuts, such as dried apricots, walnut and almond halves, and circles of crystallized citrus.
◆ After topping with fruit, glaze the cake with 2 tbsp apricot jam, heated until runny with a spoonful of boiling water.

❖ EARL GREY TEA BREAD ❖

INGREDIENTS

1¼ cups (300ml) strong, freshly brewed Earl Grey tea
½ cup (100g) dark raisins
½ cup (100g) golden raisins
½ cup (100g) candied citrus peel
oil to coat the pan
1 egg, beaten
¼ cup (50g) brown sugar
1¼ cups (150g) whole-wheat flour
1 tsp baking powder

Candied peel and strong tea give this fruit-packed tea bread a refreshing zest. Makes 10 slices.

1 In a large bowl, mix the tea, raisins, and citrus peel. Let soak overnight.
2 Preheat the oven to 350°F/180°C. Lightly oil a loaf pan with a 1lb 2oz (500g) capacity.
3 Stir the egg and sugar into the tea and fruit mixture. Sift in the flour and baking powder. Stir in the bran left in the sifter, except for 2 tablespoons, and mix well.
4 Pour the mixture into the prepared pan and bake for 1 hour, or until the edges of the bread come away from the sides of the pan and the loaf feels firm to the touch.
5 Cool the tea bread for a few minutes in the pan and then invert it onto a wire rack. Cut into slices and serve. Eat within 10 days.

NUTRITIONAL INFORMATION

Amount per serving

Calories (kcal)	158
Total fat (g)	2
% of calories	9
Sat. fat (g)	0.3
% of calories	2
Cholesterol (mg)	19
Total carb. (g)	35
Starch (g)	10
Fiber (g)	2
Protein (g)	3
Sodium (mg)	79

HEALTH LINKS

Constipation, p. 78
The body's defenses, p. 89

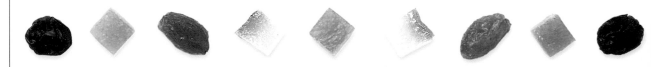

❖ OAT BRAN MUFFINS ❖

INGREDIENTS

oil to brush the muffin tins
2 tbsp sugar, optional
1½ cups (125g) oat bran
2 tsp ground cinnamon
2 tsp baking powder
6oz (175g) apple, well scrubbed
1 inch (2.5cm) strip lemon rind
3 tbsp water
¾ cup (175ml) skim milk
1 egg white
¼ cup (30g) dark raisins

These muffins are an excellent, healthier snack alternative to cookies, and this recipe has the added bonus of being gluten-free. Makes 12 muffins.

1 Preheat the oven to 400°F/200°C. Brush 12 deep muffin tins thoroughly with oil.
2 In a bowl combine the sugar, if using, oat bran, cinnamon, and baking powder.
3 In a food processor or blender, purée the apple with the lemon rind, water, milk, and egg white. Stir into the oat bran mixture with the raisins. The mixture will seem very runny at first, but it quickly thickens. Wait 5–10 minutes before using.
4 Divide the mixture among the muffin tins and bake on the top rack of the oven for 15–18 minutes, until the muffins begin to brown.
5 Invert onto a wire rack, let cool, and serve. Store in an airtight container and eat within 4 days.

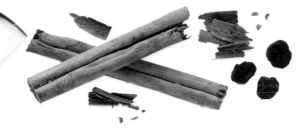

NUTRITIONAL INFORMATION

Amount per serving

Calories (kcal)	62
Total fat (g)	1
% of calories	18
Sat. fat (g)	trace
% of calories	3
Cholesterol (mg)	trace
Total carb (g)	11
Starch (g)	6
Fiber (g)	2
Protein (g)	2
Sodium (mg)	136

Rich source of iron

HEALTH LINKS

Heart health, pp. 82–5
Diabetic health, pp. 90–91
Restlessness, p. 93

VARIATIONS

◆ *Add any of the following to the mixture just before baking:*
◆ *½ cup (100g) dried cranberries or 1 cup (150g) fresh or frozen bilberries, blueberries, black currants, or chopped, pitted cherries.*
◆ *¼ cup (50g) pumpkin or sunflower seeds.*

❖ BANANA WALNUT TEA BREAD ❖

INGREDIENTS

oil to coat the pan
½ cup (75g) chopped dates
3 tbsp soft sunflower margarine
2 very ripe bananas, mashed
squeeze of lemon juice
½ cup (100ml) low-fat milk
½ cup (75g) walnut halves, roughly chopped
½ cup (75g) brown sugar
1 egg, beaten
1¾ cups (225g) all-purpose whole-wheat flour with 1½ tsp baking powder
¼ cup (25g) cocoa powder

This moist tea bread gets most of its fat and sugar from foods that also provide vitamins, minerals, and fiber. Makes 12 slices

1 Preheat the oven to 350°F/180°C. Lightly oil a 2lb (1kg) loaf pan.
2 In a large saucepan, heat ½ cup (100ml) water with the dates and bring to a boil. Remove from the heat and mash the dates roughly. Mix in the margarine.
3 Stir in the bananas, lemon juice, milk, walnuts, sugar, and egg, and mix until completely blended.
4 Sift in the flour and the cocoa powder and mix well.
5 Pour the mixture into the prepared pan and bake for about 1¼ hours, or until a skewer inserted into the center comes out clean.
6 Cool the tea bread in the pan. Eat within 2 days of baking. If you want to keep the tea bread longer, cut it into thick slices and freeze, ready for defrosting in a microwave or toaster as desired.

NUTRITIONAL INFORMATION

Amount per serving

Calories (kcal)	200
Total fat (g)	10
% of calories	43
Sat. fat (g)	2
% of calories	7
Cholesterol (mg)	17
Total carb. (g)	25
Starch (g)	12
Fiber (g)	2
Protein (g)	5
Sodium (mg)	95

Rich source of copper, phosphorus, selenium

HEALTH LINKS

Constipation, p. 78
Heart health, pp. 82–5
Nervousness, p. 93

SALSAS & DRESSINGS

FRESH-TASTING, COLORFUL relishes are today's replacements for heavy cream and butter sauces. Often almost fat-free, salsas and relishes offer another way to add vegetables and fruits to meals. Their piquant flavors add interest to the dishes they accompany, making it easy to cook with less fat and salt. Salsas enliven the plainest starchy foods and are delicious in sandwiches or baked potatoes, or on top of pasta or rice. New salad dressings contain less oil. Oils are better for your health than solid fats, but the calories are the same – and most of us are using less energy in daily life. The more often you eat salad, the more valuable it is to find a lower-fat dressing you enjoy. Flavorings such as fresh herbs and citrus juice enhance the taste of low-fat dressings. Unless specified, chop ingredients for these salsa recipes by hand: blenders make them too mushy. Knives and cutting boards that are in good condition make the job easier.

❖ PINEAPPLE SALSA ❖

INGREDIENTS

¼ lb (100g) fresh pineapple, finely diced
2 tbsp finely chopped red pepper
1 tsp finely chopped green chili pepper
3 tsp chopped fresh cilantro
2 tsp chopped fresh mint
1 tbsp lime or lemon juice

This easy relish combines some of the most sparkling flavors of the food world. It enhances any main course, notably rice dishes, poultry, and oily fish.

1 In a serving bowl, combine all of the ingredients.
2 Allow the flavors to blend for at least 10 minutes before serving.
3 Chill, covered, until ready to serve and eat within 2 days. Serve at room temperature.

NUTRITIONAL INFORMATION

Amount per serving	
Calories (kcal)	15
Total fat (g)	trace
% of calories	8
Sat. fat (g)	trace
% of calories	trace
Total carb. (g)	3
Cholesterol (mg)	0
Starch (g)	trace
Fiber (g)	trace
Protein (g)	trace
Sodium (mg)	2

Rich source of vitamin C

HEALTH LINKS

Digestion, pp. 78–9
Circulation, pp. 82–5

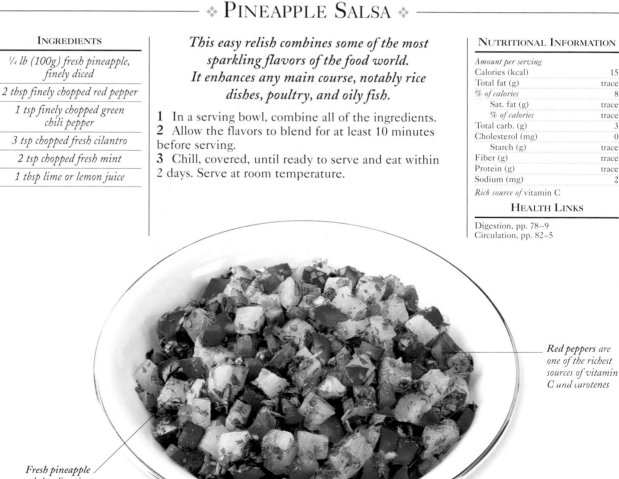

Red peppers are one of the richest sources of vitamin C and carotenes

Fresh pineapple helps digestion

❖ ZHOUG RELISH ❖

INGREDIENTS

¼ lb (120g) chopped
fresh cilantro

2 medium-hot, small chili
peppers, seeded and finely
chopped

6 garlic cloves, crushed

seeds of 6 cardamom
pods, crushed

4–5 tbsp unrefined sunflower oil

freshly ground black pepper

sea salt

Originating in the Yemen, this relish adds "zing" to rice, pasta, or potato dishes. Garlic and chili make it an ideal recipe for warding off infection. Serves 6.

1 In a small serving bowl, combine all of the ingredients and season to taste.
2 Allow flavors to blend for 5–10 minutes before serving.
3 Chill, covered, and eat within 3 days.

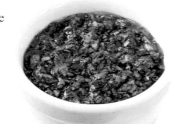

NUTRITIONAL INFORMATION

Amount per serving

Calories (kcal)	95
Total fat (g)	10
% of calories	96
Sat. fat (g)	1
% of calories	11
Cholesterol (mg)	0
Total carb. (g)	1
Starch (g)	trace
Fiber (g)	trace
Protein (g)	1
Sodium (mg)	6

Rich source of vitamin C when fresh (reduces during storage), vitamin E

HEALTH LINKS

Respiratory infections, p. 76
Digestion, pp. 78–9
Circulation and heart health pp. 82–5

❖ TOMATO SALSA ❖

INGREDIENTS

½ lb (250g) firm tomatoes

2–3 scallions or 1 shallot,
finely chopped

1 green chili pepper, seeded and
finely chopped

2 tbsp lemon or lime juice

2 tbsp chopped fresh cilantro

sea salt

VARIATIONS

◆ *Red Pepper Salsa: add a fresh or grilled red pepper, diced.*
◆ *Garlic Salsa: add 1–2 garlic cloves, crushed.*
◆ *Roast Garlic Salsa: roast 8–10 whole, peeled cloves of garlic on a sheet lightly brushed with olive oil at 350°F / 180°C for 1 hour. Halve them and add to the tomato or red pepper salsa.*
◆ *Lime Salsa: add grated zest of 1 lime.*
◆ *Cooked Salsa: cook the salsa in a spoonful of oil for a few minutes and serve hot.*

Salsa, a Mexican relish, adds a wonderful freshness to almost any dish and reduces the need for added salt.

1 Score each tomato skin with a sharp knife and place the tomatoes in a heatproof bowl. Cover them with boiling water and let stand for 1–2 minutes.
2 Lift out each tomato with a fork and remove the skin, which should peel off easily. If not, return the tomato to the hot water for a minute or two longer.
3 Chop the tomatoes and mix with all the ingredients, except the salt. Marinate for at least 20 minutes. Season to taste just before serving. Eat the same day.

NUTRITIONAL INFORMATION

Amount per serving

Calories (kcal)	14
Total fat (g)	trace
% of calories	17
Sat. fat (g)	trace
% of calories	4
Cholesterol (mg)	0
Total carb. (g)	1
Starch (g)	trace
Fiber (g)	1
Protein (g)	1
Sodium (mg)	8

Rich source of vitamin C

HEALTH LINKS

Respiratory infections, p. 76
Digestion, pp. 78–9
Circulation, pp. 82–5

Tomatoes provide one of the less common carotenes, lycopene

❖ Honey & Mustard Dressing ❖

Ingredients

1 tbsp unrefined sunflower oil

²/₃ cup (150ml) low-fat plain yogurt with active cultures

juice of 1 lemon or ¹/₂ orange

1 tsp red or white wine, optional

1 tsp coarse-grain French mustard

1 tsp cold-pressed honey

freshly ground black pepper

sea salt

Variations

◆ Add ¹/₂ garlic clove, crushed.
◆ Omit the honey and mustard, use unrefined walnut oil, and add ¹/₄ cup (25g) chopped walnuts.

This is a reduced-oil dressing that suits many salads, especially those made with cabbage and root vegetables. Makes enough to dress 2 salads.

1 In a bowl, combine the oil, yogurt, juice, wine, if using, mustard, and honey.
2 Season to taste. Store chilled and eat within 2–3 days.

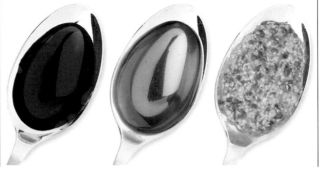

Nutritional Information

Amount per serving	
Calories (kcal)	30
Total fat (g)	2
% of calories	62
Sat. fat (g)	1
% of calories	10
Cholesterol (mg)	1
Total carb. (g)	2
Starch (g)	0
Fiber (g)	trace
Protein (g)	1
Sodium (mg)	26

Health Link

Digestion, pp. 78–9

❖ Low-Fat Hummus ❖

Ingredients

1 cup (170g) chickpeas, dry weight

¹/₄ cup (25g) sesame seeds

¹/₂ tsp coriander seeds

2 garlic cloves, crushed

juice of 1–2 lemons, to taste

2 tbsp olive oil

¹/₄ lb (120g) low-fat soft cheese

sea salt

pinch of paprika and 2 tbsp chopped fresh cilantro, to garnish

Traditionally eaten with pita bread, falafel, and salad, this lower-fat version of a classic Middle Eastern dish uses less oil and contains a higher share of chickpeas, with their notable iron and zinc level.

1 Soak the chickpeas overnight and drain.
2 Cover with fresh, cold water and bring to a boil. Reduce the heat, cover, and simmer for 1–1¹/₂ hours, until the chickpeas are cooked through.
3 Meanwhile, in an ungreased skillet, toast the sesame seeds over low heat for 3–4 minutes, then add the coriander seeds. After another minute, remove the seeds from the heat and grind them thoroughly in an electric coffee grinder.
4 Drain the chickpeas, reserving the cooking water. Transfer them to a food processor, add the ground sesame and coriander seeds, garlic, juice of 1 lemon, 1 tablespoon olive oil, and enough of the cooking water to produce a thick purée when processed.
5 Return the purée to the saucepan and stir in the soft cheese. Check the seasoning and add more lemon juice, if desired.
6 To serve, spread the hummus on a flat dish, and sprinkle with the remaining olive oil, paprika, and cilantro.

Nutritional Information

Amount per serving	
Calories (kcal)	288
Total fat (g)	17
% of calories	52
Sat. fat (g)	4
% of calories	11
Cholesterol (mg)	6
Total carb. (g)	2
Starch (g)	19
Fiber (g)	5
Protein (g)	14
Sodium (mg)	95

Rich source of copper, folic acid, iron, magnesium, phosphorus, zinc

Health Links

Circulation and heart health, pp. 82–5; Anemia, p. 85; Diabetic health, pp. 90–91

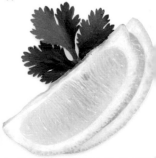

❖ CRANBERRY ORANGE RELISH ❖

INGREDIENTS

1 cup (125g) fresh or thawed frozen cranberries

2 tbsp honey

juice and zest of ½ orange

zest of ½ lemon or 1 lime

1 large apple, well scrubbed

This reduced-sugar cranberry relish is delicious eaten on its own or with meat, fish, and grain dishes.

1 Roughly chop the cranberries. Stir in 1 tablespoon of the honey and the orange juice.
2 Add the orange and lemon or lime zest.
3 Grate the apple coarsely into the mixture, stirring to prevent discoloration. Add more honey to taste.
4 Chill, covered, for at least 2 hours before serving. Eat within 3 days.

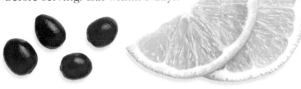

NUTRITIONAL INFORMATION

Amount per serving	
Calories (kcal)	49
Total fat (g)	trace
% of calories	2
Sat. fat (g)	0
% of calories	0
Cholesterol (mg)	0
Total carb. (g)	2
Starch (g)	0
Fiber (g)	2
Protein (g)	trace
Sodium (mg)	4

Rich source of vitamin C when fresh (reduces during storage)

HEALTH LINKS

Constipation, p. 78
Gastroenteritis, p. 79
Urinary tract infections, p. 92

❖ YOGURT & MINT DRESSING ❖

INGREDIENTS

1 cup (15g) fresh mint

1 cup (15g) fresh parsley

¼ cup (10g) fresh chives

1 cup (200ml) low-fat plain yogurt with active cultures

zest and juice of ½ lemon

½ tsp paprika

pinch of sugar, optional

freshly ground black pepper

sea salt

VARIATIONS

◆ *Substitute fresh basil, dill, fennel, cilantro, or watercress for the mint.*
◆ *Add 1 tsp dried caraway or fennel seeds, or 1 tbsp toasted, crushed linseed, sunflower, or pumpkin seeds.*

A beautiful pale green, oil-free dressing for summer salads. Makes enough to dress 2 salads.

1 Pack the herbs into a food processor or blender container. Process with just enough yogurt to make a smooth purée.
2 Transfer the purée to a bowl. By hand, stir in the remaining yogurt, the lemon zest and juice, the paprika, and the sugar, if using.
3 Season to taste. Chill until ready to serve and eat within 3 days.

NUTRITIONAL INFORMATION

Amount per serving	
Calories (kcal)	17
Total fat (g)	trace
% of calories	17
Sat. fat (g)	trace
% of calories	9
Cholesterol (mg)	1
Total carb. (g)	2
Starch (g)	trace
Fiber (g)	trace
Protein (g)	2
Sodium (mg)	24

HEALTH LINKS

Gastroenteritis, p. 79
Osteoporosis, p. 80
Yeast infections, p. 87

Fresh herbs give this salad dressing a delicate pale green color

DIRECTORY OF OTHER VALUABLE FOODS

MANY FOODS THAT ARE not featured in the *Food Profiles* section also deserve attention. These foods contribute higher-than-average amounts of nutrients per calorie and fit easily into a well-balanced diet. They widen your range of nutritious options, helping ensure all nutrients are included in your diet, and make it easier to devise meals that suit all tastes, pockets, and seasons. Some of these valuable foods, such as black raspberries, contain substances that in other foods have been linked to therapeutic benefits. But without research, we cannot assume that they share these benefits because they differ in other ways. Others, such as beets and strawberries, have been used in traditional healing but so far lack scientific backing. We can look forward to more fascinating food science.

❖ FRUITS & ❖ VEGETABLES

AVOCADO is high in vitamin E, with an average 3mg per 3½ oz (100g) flesh. It is also high in fat (10–40%, mainly monounsaturated) and calories, so enjoy it sparingly.

BEAN SPROUTS provide iron. For example, mung sprouts provide 1–2mg per 3½ oz (100g) and, if briefly stir-fried, 40mcg of folic acid.

BEETS, especially raw, are a high-class source of folic acid, providing 150mcg per 3½ oz (100g), with useful amounts of iron. Beets are surprisingly low in calories for their sweetness, but are high in oxalates and should be avoided by kidney stone sufferers.

BLACK RASPBERRIES are one of the best low-fat sources of vitamin E, with 2.4mg per 3½ oz (100g) raw berries. Like other berries of a similar color, black raspberries are rich in antho-cyanins, p. 22, but research is needed to see if these have health benefits.

CELERIAC, a form of celery, has nutrients similar to those in leafy celery, see pp. 54–5, plus more iron – 0.8mg per 3½ oz (100g) raw – and folic acid – 51mcg per 3½ oz (100g) raw. Traditionally, celeriac is shredded raw in salads, which must be coated immediately with citrus juice or dressing to avoid discoloration.

CORN provides more starch and calories than most vegetables. It is a good food for steadying blood sugar levels, since its tough cell walls and starch resist quick digestion. Despite its color, it has few carotenes and little vitamin C, but has useful amounts of iron and potassium. Baby corn, fresh or frozen, is very high in folic acid.

DRIED DATES can be treated as a more nourishing form of sugar. Date purée is a useful replacement for sugar in baking. Dried dates are a rich source of fiber and are very high in potassium and niacin, and contain some iron.

FIGS, especially dried, are well known for their laxative effect. Dried figs are rich in fiber, potassium, calcium, magnesium, and iron, and are useful as a more nourishing substitute for sugar in cooking. Early research suggests they may have some cancer-discouraging action.

GRAPES are more sugary than most fruit. All colors have a substantial level of potassium.

GUAVA provides a very high amount of vitamin C, with an average 230mg per 3½ oz (100g) flesh, although the level varies from 10–410mg.

LEEKS contain a useful amount of vitamin E, carotenes, iron, and when raw or lightly cooked, folic acid, vitamin C, and vitamin B1. They have small amounts of active constituents similar to those found in onion, see p. 36.

MANGO is a useful source of vitamin E, iron, and vitamin C when raw. Ripe mango is rich in carotenes, with about 300–3,000mcg per 3½ oz (100g) flesh.

MELON with orange flesh, as cantaloupe or Persian, contributes 800–1,900mcg carotenes per 3½ oz (100g) flesh. Servings of melon are usually large, so it is a particularly good source of carotenes. Cantaloupe may have an anticlotting action on the blood.

MUSHROOMS offer substantial amounts of potassium, niacin, pantothenic acid, and iron for very few calories. Some oriental varieties, notably shiitake, have been shown to have antiviral properties and may discourage the development of cancer.

NECTARINES provide about 37mg vitamin C per 3½ oz (100g) flesh.

PAPAYA, when raw, contains an enzyme that digests protein, so it can be used to tenderize meat and may make it more digestible. Papaya supplies about 60mg vitamin C and 800mcg carotenes per 3½ oz (100g) flesh.

PEACHES do not stand out nutritionally when fresh, apart from providing about 28mg vitamin C per 3½ oz (100g) flesh. Dried peaches, however, are very rich in potassium, with a substantial amount of iron, carotenes, and niacin.

PEARS have no outstanding nutrients, but are especially useful in cooking for sweetening sharper fruits without adding refined sugar.

POTATOES are the only starchy food apart from sweet potatoes and corn to supply a substantial amount of vitamin C. Potatoes are an outstanding source of potassium, partly because the usual portion size is at least 7oz (200g), and a useful source of vitamins B1 and B6. People prone to blood sugar fluctuations should note that potatoes cause a rapid rise in blood sugar compared with most starchy foods.

PRUNES are well known for their gentle laxative effect, and provide a useful amount of fiber and iron.

RAISINS provide a high level of potassium and iron and are useful sweeteners in cooking.

STRAWBERRIES are one of the richest sources of vitamin C, providing an average 77mg per 3½ oz (100g) fresh fruit. They are a traditional diuretic, used to relieve rheumatism or gout.

❖ NUTS & SEEDS ❖

CASHEW NUTS are high in iron, zinc, magnesium, selenium, and vitamin B1. They also contain about 50% fat, mainly monounsaturated, so enjoy them in small amounts.

HAZELNUTS contain about as much vitamin E as almonds, see pp. 70–71, and are high in vitamins B1 and B6. They are also high in fat (60%, mainly monounsaturated), so enjoy them in small amounts. Hazelnut oil is delicious and suitable for use in cold dishes and for low-temperature cooking.

PINE NUTS provide more than 13mg vitamin E per 3½ oz (100g), as well as a high level of iron, magnesium, manganese, zinc, and vitamin B1.

❖ MEAT & FISH ❖

GAME has little fat, much less than most beef, lamb, or pork, and it is mainly unsaturated fat. Hare, partridge, pigeon, grouse, and venison are higher in iron than any other meat except offal, with plenty of zinc (especially in venison), vitamins B2, B6, and B12, niacin, and pantothenate.

MEAT in very lean cuts can be a low- to medium-fat food. Beef, lamb, and any form of liver have the most absorbable form of iron and zinc, in the highest amounts. All meat supplies the complete range of B vitamins, with liver highest overall (especially folic acid), and meat is a main source of selenium. Free-range meat usually has less saturated fat than factory-reared meat. Eating a small amount of meat protein in a meal improves the amount of iron absorbed from nonmeat foods eaten at the same meal.

WHITE FISH, such as cod, haddock, flounder, and hake, have lower levels of most vitamins and minerals than oily fish, shellfish, or meat, but are high in protein, iodine, and selenium, with a useful amount of vitamins B6 and E. White fish are very low in fat and saturated fat and can improve the absorption of iron from nonmeat foods eaten at the same meal.

❖ DAIRY FOODS ❖

EGGS are high in cholesterol, but low in saturated fat. Eating 3–5 eggs a week can fit into a low-fat eating style, providing a good source of selenium and iodine, with some zinc, vitamins D and E, and the complete range of B vitamins. Eggs contain useful amounts of iron but in a form that is little absorbed. More iron is available from eggs if a food rich in vitamin C is eaten at the same meal. Egg whites, which can replace whole eggs in baking, have almost no fat, calories, minerals, or vitamins. Regularly eating raw egg whites prevents the body from making use of the B vitamin biotin. Eggs contain a small amount of estrogen, the female hormone.

HARD CHEESES, especially Parmesan, are rich in easily absorbed calcium, and in vitamin B2, protein, and zinc. Hard cheeses typically contain more than 30% saturated fat and are high in salt, so enjoy them in small amounts as a flavoring.

SOFT CHEESES, such as low-fat cottage cheese, have little calcium and zinc compared with hard cheeses, but are still very high in vitamin B2. Cottage cheese is a good source of protein.

❖ OTHER ❖

ALCOHOL Drinking 14–21 units of any form of alcohol per week substantially reduces the risk of death from stroke. Small amounts of alcoholic drinks, such as wine and liquor, can be used in place of salty or high-fat flavorings in cooking. The alcohol, but not its flavor, is removed by cooking.

COTTONSEED OIL, found in some margarines and salad dressings, is second only to wheat germ and sunflower oils for vitamin E, with 43mg per 3½ oz (100g). It is not available unrefined.

RED WINE drinkers have a lower risk of heart disease. This is thought to be due to the polyphenols, including tannins, in red grapes, see Flavonoids, p. 22. These may give red wine its antioxidant and possibly antiviral "bonus" when compared with other alcoholic drinks.

VITAMINS & MINERALS

VITAMINS AND MINERALS are essential to health, and most must be supplied by food. Deficiencies are still worldwide killers, either directly or by reducing resistance to other illnesses. In developed countries, where such a variety of food is available, it is hard to see why anyone should lack nutrients. But surveys show that a substantial proportion of people are on or under the borderline of safety, mainly because they eat badly balanced diets. A less active lifestyle means less food is needed, making it more difficult to obtain all the necessary nutrients, especially if people consume substantial amounts of sugary foods and alcohol, which supply almost no vitamins or minerals. The fewer calories eaten, the more important it is that almost every calorie carries with it some vitamins and minerals. Some people have a higher-than-average need for one or more nutrients. More of a vitamin is not always better, but we now know that for some vitamins, a higher intake can benefit people who show no signs of being deficient. For many vitamins, we can aim for optimum levels.

❖ THE NUTRIENTS WE NEED ❖

VITAMINS WE CAN STORE
Vitamins A, D, E, and B$_{12}$ can be stored in our bodies for a considerable time. Stores protect us against short-term shortages. For example, plentiful vitamin D, obtained from sunlight on our skin in summer, helps maintain our supply the following winter. But storage also means that body levels can build up and, when eaten in animal foods, even moderately excessive amounts of vitamins A and D produce ill effects. Although the body also produces vitamin A from carotenes in vegetables and fruit, eating these in large amounts does not cause vitamin A excess, nor does an excess of vitamin D result from exposure to sunlight.

In developed countries, shortages of fat-soluble vitamins A, D, E (and K, which is little stored by the body) are mainly due to poor food choice, or for vitamin D, little time spent outdoors. Some people are at risk because they absorb fat poorly, through illness or as a side effect of medication, such as cholesterol-lowering drugs or regular use of laxatives. Some vitamin A and vitamin E in food is lost due to exposure to air in storage, and strong heat during cooking, see pp. 96–7.

Fat-soluble vitamins need not come from high-fat foods: there are good low-fat sources for each one.

VITAMINS WE BARELY STORE
The B complex vitamins and vitamins C and K are little stored by the body, so daily intake is important, although the body manufactures much of the vitamin K it needs. Contact with water will wash some of these vitamins out of food – for example, in canning, soaking, or when cooking in lots of water. Food refining, exposure of cut surfaces to air and light, and prolonged heat also cause major losses. This means that the risk of deficiency is highest among people who rely on processed or overcooked food. Poor food choices and some medications are also hazards. In illness or at other times of stress, the body may benefit from higher levels of the vitamins that we barely store. B vitamins have related functions, so if you are taking a supplement, take all the B complex vitamins. To retain the maximum amount of these vitamins in food see pp. 96–7.

MINERALS
Some 15 minerals are known to be essential to human health, with a few others still under investigation. The exact amount of minerals we need to eat is even less easy to define than for vitamins because, for most minerals, the amount we absorb varies considerably according to the foods that we eat them in. We absorb some minerals less efficiently from foods high in fiber – especially when they also contain phytic acid. This is not a reason to avoid fiber, just to avoid an excess.

Certain minerals can be harmful even in moderately excessive amounts. For iron, there seems to be quite a narrow "good" body level, which is high enough to avoid the harm done by shortage, but low enough not to risk iron pro-oxidant activity, which may encourage the formation of free radicals, see Antioxidants, p. 21. A very large amount of one mineral may reduce the amount that the body can absorb of another. Such problems are unlikely if we obtain minerals from food rather than from supplements containing much larger amounts.

❖ VITAMINS ❖

MAJOR SOURCES	IMPORTANCE	EFFECTS OF SHORTAGE
VITAMIN A Available as retinol in liver, eel, fortified margarine, kidney, whole milk, and eggs. Cheese, butter, and oily fish also supply a useful amount. Also produced from carotenes in carrots, broccoli, green leafy vegetables, winter squash, sweet potatoes, red pepper, mango, pumpkins, canteloupe, and dried apricots.	Required for growth and the normal development of tissues; maintains the health of the skin and surface tissues, especially those with a mucous lining, such as the linings of the bronchial tubes. These linings are the body's first defense against infection. Vitamin A is also necessary for vision.	Vitamin A deficiency in previously well-nourished people may have no symptoms for a year or more. Early effects include poorer eyesight in low light, for example at dusk or in moonlight; dry skin; and reduced overall resistance to infection, especially in the lungs.
VITAMIN B1 (THIAMIN) Peas, wheat germ, sunflower seeds, fortified breakfast cereals, liver, yeast and yeast extract, peanuts, mycoprotein, potatoes, pork, fortified white bread, whole-grain bread, and cereal grains.	Essential for many bodily functions, including the release of energy from carbohydrates, alcohol, and fats, and the health of nerves and muscles. The more carbohydrate or alcohol is consumed, the more vitamin B1 is needed.	Early signs include irritability, failure to concentrate, depression, poor sleep, loss of appetite, and general malaise. Long-term deficiency leads to nerve damage and withering of muscles, mental confusion, and loss of memory. Outright deficiency is common among alcoholics, and prolonged deficiency is fatal.
VITAMIN B2 (RIBOFLAVIN) Liver, kidney, yogurt, milk (if packaged so that it is not exposed to light), cheese, fortified breakfast cereals, wheat germ, eggs, yeast extract, crab, mussels, winkles, oily fish, flounder, huss, whiting, mushrooms, almonds, and pumpkin seeds.	Vitamin B2 is involved in many bodily processes, especially in making energy available from food; growth in children; and the repair and maintenance of body tissues.	Early signs include sore cracks at the corners of the mouth and general malaise. Other symptoms are a form of eczema at the angles of the nose, and on the chin and genitalia, a sore, magenta-colored tongue, and red, itchy eyes. These symptoms are reversible within days and do not disable.
NIACIN (PART OF B COMPLEX) Many foods are sources of niacin, either directly or via tryptophan, a protein from which the body makes niacin. Richest sources include liver, lean meat, fortified breakfast cereals, oily fish, milk, cheese, eggs, peas, mushrooms, fish roe, green leafy vegetables, globe artichokes, asparagus, and potatoes.	Niacin comprises nicotinic acid and nicotinamide, which are both needed for the production of energy in cells. Nicotinamide is involved in enzyme processes, including fatty acid metabolism, tissue respiration, and the disposal of toxins. Niacin supplements are being researched for their usefulness in treating schizophrenia.	Deficiency is unlikely if you eat a varied diet, especially as some breakfast cereals are fortified with the vitamin. Symptoms of mild deficiency include a lack of energy, depression, and sometimes a dark red, scaly rash on the skin when it is exposed to the sun. Prolonged severe deficiency, which is very unlikely today, causes outright pellagra and death.
PANTOTHENIC ACID (PART OF B COMPLEX) Most foods except sugar, fats, and alcohol contain some pantothenic acid, or pantothenate. Rich sources include liver, whole grains, yeast extract, avocados, wheat germ, egg yolk, peanuts, walnuts, dried pears and apricots, dates, and mushrooms.	Plays a central role in making energy from fats and carbohydrates available for the production of essential substances in the body, including the production of steroid hormones and fatty acids. There is some evidence that pantothenic acid supplements can help rheumatoid arthritis, see p. 81.	Deficiency is rare, but is also hard to recognize, partly because the symptoms are vague and partly because it is usually combined with other vitamin deficiencies. Known signs include numbness and tingling sensations in the feet, headache, irritability and restlessness, dizziness, fatigue, and stomach disturbances.

MAJOR SOURCES	IMPORTANCE	EFFECTS OF SHORTAGE
VITAMIN B6 (PYRIDOXINE) Wheat germ, bananas, potatoes, turkey, fish, nuts, especially walnuts, sesame seeds, bell peppers, cruciferous vegetables, especially Brussels sprouts, cauliflower, and watercress, avocados, and fortified breakfast cereals.	Required by the body in the making of proteins, to release stored glucose, and in the production of niacin from tryptophan. All these bodily processes are necessary for growth, blood formation, and to protect against infection. The more protein that is eaten, the more vitamin B6 is required.	In theory, deficiency is rare except in some people taking certain drugs for rheumatism, tuberculosis, or high blood pressure. Symptoms include a sore mouth, depression, irritability, eczema, and sometimes inflammation of a nerve, causing pain or poor function. Supplements of 50mg per day taken for premenstrual syndrome cause side effects in many women.
BIOTIN Liver, kidney, wheat germ, nuts, oats, egg yolk, cooked dried black-eyed peas or soybeans, snow peas, globe artichokes, mushrooms, and mycoprotein. Biotin is manufactured within the body as well as being obtained from food.	Needed to make the energy from food available, for instance, for the synthesis of fats, and for the excretion of protein waste products.	The only people likely to be at risk are those who often eat more than 1–2 raw egg whites a day, which prevent the absorption of biotin. Symptoms of deficiency include nervous disturbance and seborrheic dermatitis.
FOLIC ACID Liver, yeast extract, wheat germ, green leafy vegetables, especially parsley, watercress, spinach, endive, and purple sprouting broccoli, raw beets, fortified breakfast cereals, nuts, especially peanuts, and legumes.	Needed for the production of many essential substances in the body. It is important for the role it plays with vitamin B12 in rapidly dividing cells, making genetic material (DNA) for every cell. Also required to maintain immune system function.	Mild deficiency can lead to anemia, mouth sores, a sore tongue, appetite loss, general malaise, and poor growth in children. Severe deficiency can cause mental deterioration. Women with low levels of folic acid at conception have a much higher risk of having a baby with a neural tube defect such as spina bifida. The risk is sharply reduced if women planning a pregnancy take 400mcg folic acid daily, continuing to 12 weeks, or throughout, pregnancy.
VITAMIN B12 (CYANOCOBALAMIN) Found in all animal foods, especially liver, and plant foods that contain certain algae, such as seaweed, or bacteria, such as beer; mycoprotein; fortified yeast extract; and fortified breakfast cereals.	Needed for the manufacture of genetic material (DNA and RNA), which is in every cell, vitamin B12 is also involved in the formation of red blood cells, the utilization of folic acid, and the maintenance of the protective sheaths around the nerves.	Although only minute amounts of vitamin B12 are needed for health, deficiency can slowly accumulate in people with prolonged low intake or poor absorption. The first effect of shortage is anemia, causing tiredness and loss of resistance to infection. Prolonged deficiency leads to megoblastic anemia with irreversible damage to the nervous system.
VITAMIN C (ASCORBIC ACID) Green leafy vegetables, especially raw, black currants, citrus fruits, strawberries, bell peppers, guava, tomatoes, and potatoes.	Essential for the formation and maintenance of connective tissue, wound-healing, gum health, and overall health. There is a strong connection between higher intakes of vitamin C and a lower risk of heart disease, stroke, cataracts, and some cancers.	Low levels result in deficiency symptoms within 3–4 weeks, such as increasingly poor recovery from wounds, fatigue, reduced gum health, bleeding from small blood vessels into the gums, joint pain, and poor sleep and mood. Smokers are advised to eat more. Antioxidant experts advise up to 200mg per day, far above most governments' recommended intake.

MAJOR SOURCES	IMPORTANCE	EFFECTS OF SHORTAGE
VITAMIN D (CALCIFEROLS) Vitamin D is mainly manufactured in the body when the skin is exposed to sunlight, except through glass. Few food sources: oily fish, notably herring, kippers, salmon, sardines, and trout, and, in much smaller amounts, fortified margarine, and eggs.	Needed for the absorption of calcium from food, and for calcium and phosphorus use. It therefore affects the growth and strength of bones and teeth, together with nerve and muscle health connected with calcium.	In children, there is less bone growth, muscle weakness, anemia, and a tendency to respiratory infections. Long-term shortage results in rickets, where the bones become deformed because they are too weak to bear the child's weight. In adults, shortage softens bones, causing pain, muscle weakness, and a higher risk of fractures.
VITAMIN E Nuts and seeds, especially sunflower seeds, almonds, hazelnuts, and pine nuts, and wheat germ. Sunflower spreads, sunflower oil, broccoli, green leafy vegetables, sweet potatoes, oats, avocados, and whole-grain cereals also supply a useful amount.	Two sorts of vitamin E, tocopherols and tocotrienols, are probably both needed for their antioxidant action, which protects against the harmful by-products of oxidation. The more polyunsaturated fats you eat, the more vitamin E is needed to protect them from oxidation.	Convincing evidence shows that people with lower body levels of vitamin E have a higher risk of heart attack, stroke, cataracts, and some cancers. In a few people who cannot absorb or use vitamin E adequately, a progressive neurological disorder can develop that affects the eyes, nervous system, and muscles, and causes anemia.
VITAMIN K Green leafy vegetables, notably green cabbage, Brussels sprouts, cauliflower, and spinach, liver, beans, peas, and carrots. At least half of the daily requirement is not obtained from food but is manufactured in the body.	Essential for the formation of proteins responsible for blood clotting and other functions, Vitamin K may be required for maintaining bone health.	Shortage in adults is unlikely except in people with poor fat absorption, such as sufferers of Crohn's disease, or people with severe gallstones. Lack of clotting ability causes prolonged bleeding. Newborn babies have little vitamin K, and the vitamin is often given at birth to guard against hemorrhage.

❖ MINERALS ❖

MAJOR SOURCES	IMPORTANCE	EFFECTS OF SHORTAGE
CALCIUM Milk, yogurt, hard cheese, tofu, fish eaten along with the bones, such as whitebait, canned sardines, and canned salmon, green leafy vegetables, notably purple sprouting broccoli, watercress, and spinach, okra, almonds, and hard water. Low-fat milk and yogurt have as much calcium as whole.	Essential for growth and for maintaining the strength of the bones and teeth. Calcium also controls the conduction of nerve impulses to and from the brain, and the contraction of muscles.	In the short term, there are no obvious signs of deficiency because calcium needs will be met by withdrawing it from the bones. Long-term calcium shortage, up to the age of 35–40, prevents the bones from reaching full density (peak bone mass), which may increase the risk of bone problems in old age.
CHLORIDE Table salt (sodium chloride) is about 60% chloride.	Works with sodium and potassium in regulating the body's delicate fluid balance.	Deficiency is very unlikely, except as a result of heavy and prolonged sweating or vomiting.
CHROMIUM Meat, whole-grain cereals, legumes, nuts, and seafood.	Chromium was only identified as an essential mineral about 30 years ago, and it is still not well understood. It is part of a compound needed to enable the insulin system to work. Chromium may also be involved in fat metabolism and in maintaining the structure of genetic material.	Lack of knowledge about the mineral means deficiency is rarely recognized, but it is known to cause poor glucose tolerance and raised blood cholesterol. In animals, lack of chromium causes an illness very similar to diabetes.

MAJOR SOURCES	IMPORTANCE	EFFECTS OF SHORTAGE
COPPER Shellfish, liver, wheat germ, curry powder, and whole-grain cereals.	Part of many enzymes, copper is required for a wide range of functions: blood and bone formation; production of melanin pigment of skin and hair; and energy release from food. Copper is part of the antioxidant enzyme superoxide dismutase. The use of copper bracelets to relieve rheumatism has attracted interest.	Adult deficiency is rarely recognized, but early features can include defects in heart function and anemia. More research about the effects of deficiency is in progress.
FLUORIDE Tea, seafood, and seaweed. Drinking water and other foods can supply an important amount of fluoride or almost none according to soil levels where the food or water originates.	No essential function has been found, but fluoride is useful in reducing tooth decay. It forms a compound with calcium in the bones and teeth.	Leads to a higher rate of tooth decay, although this depends on eating habits and dental hygiene as well. Even a small excess of fluoride in the body can mottle teeth permanently, so toothpaste should not be swallowed.
IODINE Seafood, especially shellfish and seaweed, and iodized salt. Levels in land-grown food vary widely, according to natural soil level variations. Milk is a source where iodine disinfectants and milk promoters are used in dairies.	Needed by the thyroid gland to produce the thyroid hormone, which regulates more than 100 enzyme systems involving the metabolic rate, growth, reproduction, and many more essential functions.	The thyroid gland (at the front of the throat) swells to try to trap more iodine from the bloodstream, forming a goiter. The metabolic rate slows, leading to sluggish physical and mental activity, weight gain, a thick neck, coarsening features, and dry hair. Severe lack manifests as mental deterioration in adults and causes low intelligence in babies.
IRON Liver, blood sausage, kidney, game, especially pigeon, venison, and partridge, whitebait, mussels, oily fish, especially sardines, dried apricots, prunes, green leafy vegetables, legumes, and tofu.	Essential for the formation of red blood cells, and so needed for the circulation because red blood cells carry oxygen around the body. Iron is also part of a number of enzymes, including some that make energy available.	Mild shortage leads to adverse effects on work capacity, intellectual performance, behavior, disease resistance, and body-temperature control. Severe shortage results in overt anemia.
MAGNESIUM Whole-grain cereals, wheat germ, nuts and seeds, shrimp, winkles, okra, chard, soybeans, tofu, and dried apricots. The absorption of magnesium is reduced when large amounts of calcium, protein, or phosphate are eaten at the same time.	Mainly present in the bones and essential for their growth, magnesium is also needed in every cell and for the functioning of some of the enzymes required for energy use. It is also required for normal calcium function.	No signs at first because magnesium is withdrawn from the bones for other uses. Later, shortage leads to muscle weakness, poor nerve–muscle interaction, lethargy, depression, irritability, and, in extreme cases, heart attack. Some researchers believe that a low intake contributes to heart attacks, but this is not established.
MANGANESE Tea, whole-grain cereals, nuts, especially pine nuts, pecans, macadamias, hazelnuts, and walnuts, green leafy vegetables, soybeans, and soy protein products, such as tofu.	Manganese is part of several essential enzymes and triggers the activities of numerous others, including antioxidant and energy-production processes.	There is no recognized deficiency disorder in humans. In animals, lack of manganese leads to abnormal offspring, and poor bone development and growth.

MAJOR SOURCES	IMPORTANCE	EFFECTS OF SHORTAGE
MOLYBDENUM Kasha, beans, wheat germ, liver, whole-grain cereals, and green leafy vegetables. Levels in food vary, according to the soil level in areas of food production.	Part of several enzymes, including mechanisms for excreting uric acid, use of iron, and DNA metabolism.	Shortage is unlikely among people eating a Western-style diet. A low intake may possibly reduce resistance to tooth decay.
PHOSPHORUS Present in all protein foods and added to many processed foods, notably carbonated beverages.	In combination with calcium, phosphorus helps maintain the strength of the bones and teeth. It is needed by the body to use energy and B vitamins from food. Phosphorus is a constituent of many essential body substances and body control mechanisms.	In adults, deficiency occurs after prolonged, regular overuse of antacids, which prevent the absorption of phosphorus. Required phosphorus is withdrawn from bones, which can become weak and painful.
POTASSIUM Fruits, notably dried fruits, such as apricots, as well as bananas and citrus fruits; vegetables, especially when raw or cooked without water, notably green leafy vegetables and potatoes; and instant coffee.	Complements sodium in regulating the fluid levels in the body. Important to help the body excrete excess sodium, which helps prevent and relieve raised blood pressure.	Potassium cannot be stored by the body, and shortage shows up immediately, causing symptoms such as feeling weak, thirsty, confused, and tired. Severe deficiency exacerbates these symptoms and leads to mental confusion and raised blood pressure, a major factor in heart attack and stroke.
SELENIUM Brazil nuts, whole-grain cereals, sunflower seeds, seafood, seaweed, and meat. Only brazil nuts, seafood, and seaweed have a reliable level. In other foods, the amount of selenium varies according to the soil level in the area of food production.	A vital part of the body's antioxidant defense system, selenium works with vitamin E and can partially replace it. Selenium may help protect against cancer, but the evidence is still inconclusive. Recent research suggests that extra selenium may improve male fertility.	No obvious symptoms, but leads to reduced fertility. Also leads to Keshan congestive heart disease, seen in areas of China where levels of selenium in the soil are low. It is cured by selenium supplements. Lack of selenium is also linked to reduced antioxidant protection, see p. 21.
SODIUM More than two-thirds of the sodium we eat comes from the salt and sodium preservatives already added to the food we buy, for example, meat products and delicatessen meats, bacon, cheese, bread, baking powder, potato chips, soups, pickles, breakfast cereals, and canned vegetables. Sodium is also obtained from the salt added to cooking, and is naturally present in food and water.	Sodium is essential in small amounts for regulating the body's balance of fluid, in conjunction with potassium and chloride.	Deficiency is very unlikely, and almost everyone in industrialized countries has an excessive intake of sodium. This can lead to fluid retention and raised blood pressure. Only being in intense hot weather or sweating copiously will cause deficiency symptoms such as thirst, cramps, or muscle weakness.
ZINC Oysters and other shellfish, lean meat, pumpkin seeds, milk, hard cheese, yogurt, nuts, sunflower seeds, beans, and whole-wheat bread.	Required for the health of the immune system, normal growth, tissue formation, male sexual maturation, and the action of various enzymes. More zinc is needed when new tissue must be formed, for example, when recovering from surgery or burns, or during wound-healing.	Leads to loss of appetite, an impaired sense of taste and smell, slow wound-healing, poor hair growth, dermatitis, lower resistance to illness, poor growth, and complications during pregnancy.

❖ DAILY AMOUNTS FOR GOOD HEALTH ❖

Eating the amounts of vitamins and minerals shown below should provide enough, or more than enough, for almost everyone in good health. These US Daily Recommended Amounts allow for individuals with higher needs (but not for needs during illness).

VITAMIN A
Men 15+	1,000mcg
Women 11+	800mcg

⸱⸱⸱⸱⸱⸱ *Important note* ⸱⸱⸱⸱⸱⸱
Excess retinol is harmful: be cautious when taking supplements. Eating plenty of foods rich in carotenes is safe and has benefits beyond ensuring vitamin A, see p. 22.

VITAMIN B1
Men 15+	1.2mg
Women 15+	1.0mg

VITAMIN B2
Men 19–50	1.7mg
Men 50+	1.4mg
Women 15+	1.2mg

NIACIN
Men 19–50	19mg
Women 11–50	15mg
Men 50+	15mg
Women 50+	13mg

PANTOTHENIC ACID
Men / Women 11+	4–7mg

VITAMIN B6
Men 19+	2mg
Women 19+	1.6mg

BIOTIN
Men / Women 11+	30–100mcg

FOLIC ACID
Men 15+	200mcg
Women 15+	180mcg

⸱⸱⸱⸱⸱⸱ *Important note* ⸱⸱⸱⸱⸱⸱
Women planning a pregnancy should take 400 mcg folic acid daily, continuing to 12 weeks, or throughout, pregnancy.

VITAMIN B12
Men 15+	2.0mcg
Women 15+	1.5mcg

VITAMIN C
Men / Women 15+	60mg

⸱⸱⸱⸱⸱⸱ *Important note* ⸱⸱⸱⸱⸱⸱
Smokers are advised to eat 80mg. More than 1g per day may cause diarrhea and an increased risk of kidney stones.

VITAMIN D
Men / Women 25+	5mcg

⸱⸱⸱⸱⸱⸱ *Important note* ⸱⸱⸱⸱⸱⸱
Anyone who rarely exposes any skin to outdoor light is advised to take vitamin D supplements. To obtain sufficient quantities from food alone, a weekly intake of about 1lb (450g) of the richest food source, herring or kippers, would be needed.

VITAMIN E
Men 11+	10mg
Women 11+	8mg

⸱⸱⸱⸱⸱⸱ *Important note* ⸱⸱⸱⸱⸱⸱
Official recommendations for vitamin E intake are far lower than the 40–60mg a day suggested by some antioxidant experts as desirable for people at risk of degenerative disease. To obtain this amount from food requires a major shift toward sunflower or wheat germ products.

VITAMIN K
Men 19–24	75mcg
Women 19–24	60mcg
Men 25+	80mcg
Women 25+	65mg

CALCIUM
Both sexes
11–24	1,200mg
25+	800mg

⸱⸱⸱⸱⸱⸱ *Important note* ⸱⸱⸱⸱⸱⸱
Taking high-potency calcium supplements may reduce the quantity of magnesium, iron, and zinc absorbed by the body and may encourage kidney stones.

CHLORIDE
Men / Women 11+	750mg

CHROMIUM
There are no set recommended amounts because of lack of knowledge, but the estimated need for adults is at least 50–200mcg per day. The more sugar eaten, the more chromium is needed.

COPPER
Men / Women 15+	1.5–3mg

⸱⸱⸱⸱⸱⸱ *Important note* ⸱⸱⸱⸱⸱⸱
High levels of copper are toxic, but do not occur from food unless copper saucepans are used in cooking.

FLUORIDE
There is no recommended intake because the amount naturally present in food and water varies so widely in different areas. People who live in low-fluoride areas are advised to use (but not swallow) fluoride toothpaste rather than take supplements, which risk overdose.

IODINE
Men / Women 11+	150mcg

⸱⸱⸱⸱⸱⸱ *Important note* ⸱⸱⸱⸱⸱⸱
People who live in areas with low soil iodine are at higher risk of shortage.

IRON
Men 19+	10mg
Women 15–50	15mg
Women 50+	10mg

⸱⸱⸱⸱⸱⸱ *Important note* ⸱⸱⸱⸱⸱⸱
Women with high menstrual blood loss may need extra iron. Do not take iron supplements unless a test has shown your hemoglobin level to be low.

MAGNESIUM
Men 19+	350mg
Women 19+	280mg

MANGANESE
There are no set recommended amounts, but the estimated need for adults is 2–9mg.

MOLYBDENUM
There are no set recommended amounts, but the US Food and Nutrition Board suggests 500mcg.

PHOSPHORUS
Men / Women 25+	800mg

POTASSIUM
Men / Women 15+	2,000mg (minimum amount)

SELENIUM
Men 19+	70mcg
Women 19+	55mcg

⸱⸱⸱⸱⸱⸱ *Important note* ⸱⸱⸱⸱⸱⸱
Selenium is toxic at a level of 3–6mg per day.

SODIUM
Men / Women 11+	500mg

ZINC
Men 11+	15mg
Women 11+	12mg

⸱⸱⸱⸱⸱⸱ *Important note* ⸱⸱⸱⸱⸱⸱
Zinc supplements should not be taken regularly. Too much zinc reduces the absorption of iron and copper.

BIBLIOGRAPHY

Bingham, Dr. S. *The Everyman Companion to Food and Nutrition,* Dent, London, 1987.

Committee on Medical Aspects of Food Policy Report. *Nutritional Aspects of Cardiovascular Disease,* HMSO, London, 1994.

Garrow, J. S. and James, W. P. (eds). *Human Nutrition and Dietetics,* 9th edition, Churchill Livingstone, New York, 1993.

Grieve, M. *A Modern Herbal,* Dover, New York, 1972.

McGee, H. *On Food and Cooking,* Collier Books, Macmillan Publishing Co., New York, 1984.

Messegue, M. *Health Secrets of Plants and Herbs,* Pan, London, 1981.

Mills, S. Y. *Out of the Earth,* Viking, New York, 1991.

Werbach, Dr. M. R. *Healing Through Nutrition,* HarperCollins, New York, 1995.

World Health Organization Study Group Report. *Diet, Nutrition and the Prevention of Chronic Diseases,* Geneva, 1990.

Workman, E. et al. *Arthritis Food Tolerance Book,* 1986.

KEY REFERENCES

Dietary Reference Values
"Dietary reference values for food energy and nutrients for the United Kingdom," report of Committee on Medical Aspects of Food Policy (COMA), pub. Her Majesty's Stationery Office (HMSO), 1991.
"Health of the nation" report, Department of Health, UK (HMSO), 1992.
"International tables of glycemic index." *Am J Clin Nutr* (1995); 62:871S–93S.

ALMOND
Abbey, M. et al. "Partial replacement of saturated fatty acids with almonds or walnuts lowers total plasma cholesterol and low-density-lipoprotein cholesterol." *Am J Clin Nutr* (1991); 59(5):995–9.
2 large-scale studies, i.e.
Fraser, G. E. et al. "A possible protective effect of nut consumption on risk of coronary heart disease: the Adventist Health Study." *Arch Intern Med* (1992); 152:1416–24.
See also Antioxidants, Essential fatty acids.

ANTIOXIDANTS
Albanes, D. et al. "The effect of vitamin E and beta-carotene on the incidence of lung cancer and other cancers in male smokers." *NE J Med* (1994); 330(15):1029–35.
Colditz, G. A. et al. "Increased green and yellow vegetable intake and lowered cancer deaths in an elderly population." *Am J Clin Nutr* (1985); 11(1):32–6.
Diplock, A. "Antioxidants and disease prevention" (review). *Molec Aspects Med* (1994); 15:293–376.

Gey, K. F. "Inverse correlation between the plasma level of antioxidant vitamins and the incidence of ischemic heart disease in cross-sectional epidemiology." *Agents and Actions* (1987); 222:3–4.
Gey, K. F. et al. "Poor plasma status of carotene and vitamin C is associated with higher mortality from ischemic heart disease and stroke: Basel Prospective study." *Clin Invest* (1993); 71:3–6.
Jacques, P. et al. "Antioxidant status in those with and without cataract." *Arch Opthalmol* (1988); 106:337.
Kardinaal et al. "Antioxidants in adipose tissue and risk of myocardial infarction: the EURAMIC study." *The Lancet* (1993); 342:1379–84.
Kune, G. A. et al. "Diet, alcohol, smoking, serum beta-carotene, and vitamin A in male nonmelanocytic skin cancer patients and controls." *Nutr Cancer* (1992); 18(3):237–44.
Manson, J. E. et al. "Antioxidant vitamin consumption and incidence of stroke in women." *Circulation* (1993); 87:678.
Momas, I. et al. "Relative importance of risk factors in bladder carcinogenesis: some new results about Mediterranean habits." *Cancer Causes Control* (1991); 5(1):326–32.
Riemersma, R. A. et al. "Risk of angina pectoris and plasma concentrations of vitamins A, C and E and carotene." *The Lancet* (1991); 5 Jan.
Seddon, J. M. et al. "Dietary carotenoids, vitamins A, C and E, and advanced age-related macular degeneration." *JAMA* (1994); 272(18):1413–20.
Veris. "Vitamin E Research Summary" (September 1991).

5325 South Ninth Avenue, LaGrange, Ill 60525.
Woodall, A. A. et al. "Dietary supplementation with carotenoids: effects on a-tocopherol levels and susceptibility of tissues to oxidative stress." *BJ Nutr* (1996); 76:307–317.

APPLE
Friedman, M. et al. "Effect of heating on mutagenicity of fruit juices in the Ames test." *J Ag and Food Chem* (1990); March:740–3.
Konowalchuk, J. et al. "Antiviral effect of apple beverages." *App and Environ Microbiol* (1978); Dec:798–801.
Sable-Amplis, R. et al. "Further studies on the cholesterol-lowering effect of apple in humans: biochemical mechanisms involved." *Nutr Res* (1983); 3:325–8.
See also Fiber.

APRICOT
See Antioxidants, Fiber, Dietary Reference Values.

ARTICHOKE
Gebhardt, R. "Protective antioxidant activity of extracts of artichokes in hepatic cells." *Elsevier Science BV,* Amsterdam, Netherlands.
Wojcicki, J. et al. "Effect of preparation Cynarex on the blood serum lipids level of the workers exposed to chronic action of carbon disulfide." *Elsevier Science BV,* Amsterdam, Netherlands.

ASPARAGUS
Dalvi, S. S. et al. "Effect of *Asparagus racemosus* (Shatavari) on gastric emptying time in normal healthy volunteers." *J Postgrad Med* (1990); 36(2):91–4.

Grieve, M. *A Modern Herbal,* Rev. ed. Tiger Books, London, 1992.

BANANA
Several studies, i.e.
Spring, B. et al. "Carbohydrates, tryptophan and behaviour." *Psychological Bulletin* (1987); 102(2):234–256.
Wurtman, R. J. "Ways that foods can affect the brain." *Nutrition Review/Supplement* (1986); May:2–5.
See also Fiber.

BEANS & LENTILS
Jenkins, D. J. A. et al. "Leguminous seeds in the dietary management of hyperlipidemia." *Am J Clin Nutr* (1983); 38:567–73.
See also Fiber, Dietary Reference Values.

BILBERRY
Several studies, i.e.
Ghiringhelli, C. et al. "Capillarotropic activity of anthocyanosides in high doses in phlebopathic stasis." *Min Cardioangiol* (1978); 26:255–76.
Grismond, G. L. "Treatment of pregnancy-induced phlebopathies." *Min Ginecol* (1981); 33:221–30.
Mian, E. et al. "Anthocyanosides and the walls of micro-vessels." *J Minerva Med* (1977); 68(52):3565–81.
Ofek, I. et al. "Anti-escherichia adhesion activity of cranberry and blueberry juices." *NE J Med* (1991); 324:1599.
Pennarola, R. et al. "The therapeutic action of the anthocyanosides in microcirculatory changes due to adhesive-induced polyneuritis." *Gazz Med Ital* (1980); 139:485–91.

Scharrer, A. et al. "Anthocyanosides in the treatment of retinopathies." *Klin Monatsbl Augenheilkd* (1981); 178:386–9. *See also* Flavonoids.

BLACK CURRANT
Kyerematen, G. et al. "Preliminary pharmacological studies of Pecarin, a new preparation from *Ribes nigrum* fruits." *Acta Pharm Suececa* (1986); 23(2):101–6. *See also* Bilberry re. anthocyanins, Flavonoids.

BLUEBERRY
See Bilberry.

BROCCOLI
See Antioxidants, Other special properties.

CABBAGE
Cheney, G. et al. "Anti-peptic ulcer dietary factor." *J Am Diet Assoc.* (1950); 26:668–72.
Michnovicz, J. J. et al. "Induction of estradiol metabolism by dietary indole-3-carbinol in humans." *J Natl Cancer Inst* (1990); 82:947–9.
Singh, G. B. et al. "Effect of *Brassica oleracea var. capitata* in the prevention and healing of experimental peptic ulceration." *Ind J Med Res* (1962); 50(5):741.
See also Antioxidants, Cruciferous vegetables, Other special properties.

CARROT
Beuchat, L. R. et al. "Inhibitory effects of raw carrots on *Listeria monocytogenes*." *App and Environ Microbiol* (1990); 56(6):1734–42.
Nguyen, T. C. et al. "The lethal effect of carrot on listeria species." *J App Bacteriol* (1991); 70(6):479–88.
Robertson et al. "The effect of raw carrot on serum lipids and colon function." *Am J Clin Nutr* (1979); 32:1889–92.
33 studies on cancer, i.e.
Pisani, P. et al. "Carrots, green vegetables and lung cancer: a case-control study." *Int J Epidemiol* (1986); 15(4):463–8.
Steinmetz, K. A. et al. Review, *see* Other special properties.
See also Antioxidants, Other special properties.

CELERY
Grieve, M. *A Modern Herbal.* Rev. ed. Tiger Books, London, 1992.
Kulshrestha, V. K. et al. "A study of central pharmacological activity of alkaloid fraction of *Apium*

graveolens Linn." *Ind J Med Res* (1970); 58, Jan 1.
Le, O. T. et al. "Mechanisms of the hypotensive effect of 3-normal-butyl phthalide (BUPH)." *Clin Res* (1992); 40(2):326.
Mills, S. Y. *Dictionary of Modern Herbalism.* Thorsons, London, 1985.
Tsi, D. et al. "Effects of aqueous celery (*Apium graveolens*) extract on lipid parameters of rats fed a high-fat diet." *Planta Med*, Germany (1995); 61/1:18–21.

CHERRY
Blau, L. W. "Cherry diet control for gout and arthritis." *Texas Rep Bio Med* (1950); 8:309–11.

CHICKEN LIVER
Fortes, C. "Aging, zinc and cell-mediated immune response." *Aging Clin Exp Res* (1995); 7:75–6.

CHILI PEPPER
Buck, S. et al. "The neuropharmacology of capsaicin: review of some recent observations." *Pharm Review* (1986); 38:179–226.
Wang, J. P. et al. "Anti-platelet effect of capsaicin." *Thrombosis Research* (1984); 36:497–507.
Ziment, I (ed). *Practical Pulmonary Disease.* John Wiley & Sons, New York, 1983.

CITRUS FRUITS
Several studies, i.e.
Baekay, P. A. et al. "Grapefruit pectin inibits hypercholesterolemia and atherosclerosis in miniature swine." *Clin Cardiol* (1988); 11(9):595–600.
Galati, E. M. et al. "Biological effects of hesperidin, a citrus flavonoid: anti-inflammatory and analgesic activity." *Il Farmaco* (1994); 49(11):709–12.
Parker, R. and Root, M. Paper on citrus and cancer presented at *2nd International Conference on Antioxidant Vitamins and Beta-Carotene*, Berlin, Germany, 1994.
Tanizawa, H. et al. "Studies of natural antioxidants in citrus species 1. Determination of antioxidative activities of citrus fruits." *Chem Pharm Bull* (1992); 40(7):1940–2.
Wattenberg, L. W. et al. "Inhibition of carcinogenesis by some minor dietary constitutents." *Princess Takamatsu Symp.* (1985); 16:193–203.
See also Flavonoids.

CRANBERRY
Konowalchuk, J., Speirs, J. I. "Antiviral effect of commercial juices and beverages." *App and Envir Microbiol* (1978); 35:1219–29.
Light, et al. "Urinary ionised calcium in urolithiasis." *Urology* (1973); 1:67–70.
Schmidt, D. R., Sobota, A. E. "An examination of the anti-adherence activity of cranberry juice on urinary and nonurinary bacterial isolates." *Microbios* (1988); 55:173–81.
Sobota, A. E. "Inhibition of bacterial adherence by cranberry juice: potential use for the treatment of urinary tract infections." *J Urol* (1984); 131:1013–6.
Swartz, J. H., Medrek, T. F. "Antifungal properties of cranberry juice." *App Microbiol* (1968); 16:1527–7.
Zafriri et al. "Inhibitory activity of cranberry juice on adherence of type 1 and type P fimbriated *Escherichia coli* to eucaryotic cells." *Antimicrob Agents Chemother* (1989); 33:92–8.
See also Bilberry.

CRUCIFEROUS VEGETABLES
Beecher, C. W. "Cancer preventive properties of varieties of *Brassica oleracea*: a review." *Am J Clin Nutr* (1994); 59(5):1166S–70S.
Jongen, W. M. F. "Glucosinolates in brassica: occurrence and significance as cancer-modulating agents." *BJ Nutr* (1996); 55:1B:433–446.
See also Antioxidants, Other special properties.

ESSENTIAL FATTY ACIDS
Simopoulos, A. P. "Omega-3 fatty acids in health and disease and in growth and development" (review). *Am J Clin Nutr* (1991); 54:438–63.
Unsaturated fatty acids report, British Nutrition Foundation, London, Rev. ed. 1994.

FENNEL
Albert-Puleo, M. "Fennel and anise as estrogenic agents." *J Ethnopharm* (1980); 2:337–44.
Dodds, E. C. et al. "A simple aromatic oestrogenic agent with an activity of the same order as that of oestrone." *Nature* (1937); April 10:627–8.
Forster, H. B. et al. "Antispasmodic effects of some

medicinal plants." *Planta Med*, Germany (1980); 40(4):303–19.
Grieve, M. *A Modern Herbal.* Rev. ed. Tiger Books, London, 1992.
13th-century herbal: *Macer Floridus de Viribus Herbarum.* Author not known.

FIBER
Many studies, i.e.
Anderson, J. W. et al. *Soluble fiber: hypocholesterolemic effects and proposed mechanisms. Dietary fiber: chemistry, physiology, and health effects.* New York: Plenum Press, 1990; 339–347.
Haber, G. B. et al. "Depletion and disruption of dietary fibre. Effects on satiety, plasma-glucose and serum insulin." *The Lancet* (1977); ii:679–82.

FLAVONOIDS
Hertog, M. G. L. "Epidemiological evidence on potential health properties of flavonoids." *BJ Nutr* (1996); 55:1B:385–397.
Knekt, P. et al. "Flavonoid intake and coronary mortality in Finland: a cohort study." *BMJ* (1996); 312:478–81.

GARLIC
Many studies, i.e.
Adetumbi, M. A. et al. "*Allium sativum*: a natural antibiotic." *Med. Hypotheses* (1983); 12(3):227–37.
Barrie, S. A. et al. "Effects of garlic oil on platelet aggregation, serum lipids and blood pressure in humans." *J Orthomol Med* (1987); 2(1):15–21.
Ernst, E. "Cardiovascular effects of garlic (*Allium sativum*): a review." *Pharmatherapeutica* (1987); 5(2):83–9.
Hughes, B. G. et al. "Antimicrobial effects of garlic." *Phytother Res* (1991); 5:154–8.
Lau, B. H. S. et al. "*Allium sativum* (garlic) and cancer prevention" (review). *Nut Res* (1990); 10:937–48.
Warshafsky, S. et al. "Effect of garlic on total serum cholesterol." *Ann Intern Med* (1993); 119:599–605.
Weber, N. D. et al. "In vitro virucidal effects of *Allium sativum* (garlic) extract and compounds." *Planta Med*, Germany (1992); 58:417–23.
You, W. C. et al. "Allium vegetables and reduced risk of stomach cancer." *J Natl Cancer Inst* (1989); 81(2):162–4.
See also Onion, Other special properties.

GINGER

Grontved, A. et al. "Ginger root against seasickness: a controlled trial on the open sea." *Acta Otol* (1988); 105:45–9.

Mowrey, D. et al. "Motion sickness, ginger and psychophysics." *The Lancet* (1982); 1:655–657.

Srivastava, K. C. et al. "Ginger (*Zingiber officinale*) in rheumatism and muscoskeletal disorders." *Med Hypothesis* (1992); 39:342–8.

Suekawa, M. et al. "Pharmacological studies on ginger l." *J Pharm Dyn* (1984); 7:836–48.

Yamahara, J. et al. "Gastrointestinal motility enhancing effect of ginger and its active constituents." *Chem Pharm Bulletin* (1990); 38(2):430–1.
See also Onion.

HONEY

Al Somal, N. et al. "Susceptibility of *Helicobacter pylori* to the antibacterial activity of manuka honey." *J R Soc Med* (1994); 87:9–112.

Ali, A. T. M. M. et al. "Natural honey prevents indomethacin and ethanol-induced gastric lesions in rats." *Saudi Med J* (1990); 11:275–9.

Haffejee, I. E. et al. "Honey in the treatment of infantile gastroenteritis." *BMJ* (1985); 290:1866–7.

Jeddar, A. et al. "The antibacterial action of honey." *South Africa Medical Journal* (1985); 67(7):257–8.

Peterson, W. *American Bee Journal* (1969)

Russell, K. M. "The antibacterial properties of honey." University of Waikate, Hamilton, New Zealand (1983).

LETTUCE & SALAD GREENS

Crosby, D. G. *J Fd Sc* (1963); 28:347.

Grieve, M. *A Modern Herbal*, Rev. ed. Tiger Books, London, 1992.
See also Antioxidants.

LINSEED

Cunane, S. C. et al. "High alpha-linolenic acid flaxseed (*Linum usitatissimum*): some nutritional properties in humans." *B J Nut* (1993); 69:443–53.

Jens, R. et al. "Results of a study investigating the use of a combination of linseed and whey for treating chronic constipation in 114 patients in the Vienna area." *Der Praktische Arzt* (1981); 35:80–96.

Wirths, W. et al. "Fiber-rich snacks with reference to their effect on the digestive activity and blood lipids of the elderly." *Z Gerontol* (1985); 18(2):107–10.
See also Essential fatty acids, Fiber, Phytoestrogens.

OATS

Many studies, i.e.
Anand and Becker, H. et al. "Biologie, Chemie und Pharmakologie pflanzlicher sedativa." *Zeitschrift für phytother* (1984); 5:817–23.

Anderson, J. *Dr. Anderson's HCF Diet*. Martin Dunitz, London, 1984.

Anderson, J. et al. "Hypocholesterolemic effects of oatbran or bean intake for hypercholesterolemic men." *Am J Clin Nutr* (1984); 6:1146.

Janatuinen, E. K. et al. "A comparison of diets with and without oats in adults with celiac disease." *NE J Med* (1995); 333:1033–37.

Turnbull, W. H., Leeds, A. R. "Reduction of total and LDL-cholesterol in plasma by rolled oats." *J Clin Nutr and Gastroent* (1987); 2(4).

Valle-Jones, J. C. "Open study of oatbran meal biscuits in treatment of constipation in the elderly." *Curr Med Res Opin* (1985); 10:716–20.

Van Horn, L. V. et al. "Serum lipid response to oat product intake with a fat-modifed diet." *J Am Dietetic Ass* (1986); 6:759–64.

OILY FISH

Hundreds of studies, i.e.
Allen, B. R. "Fish oil in combination with other therapies in the treatment of psoriasis."

Bjorneboe, A. et al. "Effect of dietary supplementation with eicosapentaenoic acid in the treatment of atopic dermatitis." *B J Dermat* (1987); 117:463–9.

Bonaa, K. H. et al. "Effect of EPA and DHA acids on blood pressure in hypertension." *NE J Med* (1990); 322:795–801.

Burr, M. L. et al. "Effects of changes in fat, fish and fibre intakes on death and myocardial infarction: diet and reinfarction trial (DART)." *The Lancet* (1989); ii:757–61.

Fuhrer, H. et al. "Diet and fatty acids: can fish substitute for fish oil?" *Clin and Exper Rheumatology* (1991); 9:403–6.

Kremer, J. M. et al. *Different doses of fish-oil fatty acid ingestion in active rheumatoid arthritis: a prospective study of clinical and immunological parameters*. Plenum Press, New York, 1989; 343–50.

Kromhout, D. et al. "The inverse relation between fish consumption and 20-year mortality from coronary heart disease." *NE J Med* (1985); 312(19):1205–9.

Simopoulos, A. P. et al. "Health effects of n-3 polyunsaturated fatty acids in seafoods." *World Rev Nutr Diet* (1991); 66: 436–45.

Singer, P. et al. "Lipid and blood pressure lowering effect of eicosapentaenoic acid-rich diet." *Biomedica Biochem* (1984); Acta 43(8/):S421.
See also Essential fatty acids.

ONION

Several studies, i.e.
Dorsch, W. et al. "Antiallergic and antiasthmatic effects of onion extracts." *Folia Allergol Immunol Clin* (1984); 30:17.

Elnima, E. I. et al. "The antimicrobial activity of garlic and onion extracts." *Pharmazie* (1983); 38(11):747–8.

Gupta, N. N. et al. "Effect of onion on serum cholesterol, blood coagulation factors and fibrinolytic activity in alimentary lipemia." *Ind J Med Res* (1966); 54(1):18–53.

Kawakishi, S. et al. "New inhibitor of platelet aggregation in onion oil." *The Lancet* (1988); Aug. 6:330.

Louria, D. B. et al. "Onion extract in treatment of hyertension and hyperlipidemia: a preliminary communication." *Curr Ther Res* (1985); 37(1):127–31.

Srivastava, K. C. "Effects of aqueous extracts of onion, garlic and ginger on platelet aggregation and metabolism of arachidonic acid in the blood vascular system: in vitro study." *Prostaglandins Med* (1984); 13:227–35.

Wagner, H. et al. "Antiasthmatic effects of onions: inhibition of 5-lipoxygenase and cyclooxygenase in vitro by thiosulfinates and cepaenes." *Prost Leuk and EFAs* (1990); 39:59–62.
See also Other special properties.

OTHER SPECIAL PROPERTIES

Over 100 studies, i.e.
Gillman, M. W. et al. "Protective effect of fruits and vegetables on development of stroke in men." *JAMA* (1995); 273(14):1113.

Helser, M. A. et al. "Influence of fruit and vegetable juices on the endogenous formation of N-nitrosoproline and N-nitrosothiazolidine-4-carboxylic acid in humans on controlled diets." *Carcinogenesis* (UK) (1992); 13/12:2277–80.

Howe, G. R. et al. "Dietary factors and risk of breast cancer: combined analysis of 12 case-control studies." *J Natl Cancer Inst* (1990); 83:561–9.

Potter, J. "Plant foods and cancer risk." *The Caroline Walker Lecture* (1994). Pub. Caroline Walker Trust, London.

Rhodes, M. J. C. "Physiologically active substances in plant foods: an overview." *BJ Nutr* (1996); 55:1B:371–384.

Steinmetz, K. A. et al. "Vegetables, fruit and cancer. I. Epidemiology. II. Mechanisms." *Cancer Causes and Control* (1991a); 2: 325–357 and (1991b); 2:427–42.

PARSLEY

Ohyama, S. et al. "Ingestion of parsley inhibits the mutagenicity of male human urine following consumption of fried salmon." *Mutat Res* (1987); 192(1):7–10.

Zheng, G. Q. et al. "Inhibition of benzo[a]pyrene-induced tumorigenesis by myristicin, a volatile aroma constituent of parsley leaf oil." *Carcinogenesis* (1992); 13(10):1921–3;
See also Antioxidants.

PEAS

Smidt, L. J. et al. "Influence of thiamin supplementation of the health and general well-being of an elderly Irish population with marginal thiamin deficiency." *J Gerontol* (1991); 46:M16–22.
See also Fiber, Phytoestrogens.

PHYTOESTROGENS

Adlercreutz, H. et al. "Diet and breast cancer." *Acta Oncolog* (1992); 31(2):175–181.

Cassidy, A. "Physiological effects of phyto-oestrogens in relation to cancer and other human health risks." *Proc Nutr Soc* (1996); 55:1B:399–417.

Cassidy, A. et al. "Biological effects of isoflavones in young women: importance of the chemical compostion of soya bean products." *BJ Nutr* (1995); 74:587–601.

Erdman, J. W. et al. "Short-term effects of soybean isoflavones on bone in postmenopausal women." *2nd International Symposium on Soy, American Soybean Assoc.*, Brussels, 1996.

Murkies, A. L. et al. "Dietary flour supplementation decreases post-menopausal hot flushes: effect of soy and wheat." *Maturitas* (1995); 21:189–195.

Rose, D. P. "Dietary fiber, phytoestrogens and breast cancer." *Nutrition* (1992); 8:1:47–51.

Wilcox, G. et al. "Oestrogenic effects of plant foods in post-menopausal women." *BMJ* (1990); 301, October 20:905–6.

PINEAPPLE

Hundreds of studies, i.e.

Chen, G. R. "In vitro and in vivo studies on the effect of bromelain on cholesterol-protein binding." *Diss Abstr Inter* (1975); B35:6013.

Cohen, G. "Bromelain therapy in rheumatoid arthritis." *Penn Med J* (1964); 127–31.

Felton, G. E. "Fibrinolytic and antithrombotic action of bromelain may eliminate thrombosis in heart patients." *Medical Hypoth* (1980); 1123–33.

Heinecke, R. M. et al. "Effect of bromelain (Ananase) on human platelet aggregation." *Experientia* (1972); 28:844.

Nieper, H. A. "Wirkung von Bromelain auf Koronare Herzkrankheit und Angina Pectoris." *Erfahrungsheilkunde* (1978); 5:274–5.

Taussig, S. J. et al. "Bromelain, the enzyme complex of pineapple (*Ananas comosus*) and its clinical application: an update." *J Ethnopharm* (1988); 22:191–203.

PUMPKIN SEEDS

Carbin, B. E. et al. "Treatment of benign prostatis hyperplasia with phytosterols." *B J Urol* (1990); 66(6):639–11.

Suphakarn, V. S. et al. "The effect of pumpkin seeds on oxalcrystalluria and urinary compositions of children in hyperendemic area." *Am J Clin Nutr* (1987); 15(1):115–21.

RED PEPPER

See Antioxidants, Other special properties.

SEAWEED

Several studies, i.e.

Eskin, B. et al. "Mammary gland dysplasia in iodine deficiency." *JAMA* (1967); 200.691–5.

Ghent, W. R. et al. "Elemental iodine supplementation in clinical breast dysplasia." *Abstract Proc Annu Meet Am Assoc Cancer Res* (1986); 27:189.

Teas, J. "Dietary intake of laminaria, a brown seaweed, and breast cancer prevention." *Nutrition Cancer* (1983); 4(3):217–22.

Teas, J. et al. "Dietary seaweed (*Laminaria*) and mammary carcinogenesis in rats." *Cancer Res* (1984); 44(7):2758–61.

Yamamoto, I. et al. "Antitumour activity of edible marine algae." *Hydrobiologica* (1984); 116/117:145–8.

SHELLFISH

Fraker, P. J. et al. "Interrelationship between zinc and immune function." *Fed Proc* (1986); 45:1474–9.

Gibson, R. G. et al. "Perna canaliculus in the treatment of arthritis." *The Practitioner* (1980); 224:955–60.

Turnbull, A. J. et al. "Zinc – a precious metal." *Brit Nutritional Foundation Bulletin* (1989); Jan: 23–35.

SOYBEAN

Many studies, i.e.

Barnes, S. et al. "Chemoprevention by powdered soy bean chips (PSC) of mammary tumors in rats." *Breast Cancer Res Treat* (1988); 12:128.

Clarkson, T. B. et al. "Estrogenic soybean isoflavones and chronic disease." *TEM* (1995); 6:11–16.

Harding, C. et al. "Dietary soy supplementation is oestrogenic in menopausal women." *2nd International Symposium on Soy, American Soybean Assoc.*, Brussels, 1996.

Lee, H. P. et al. "Dietary effects on breast-cancer risk in Singapore." *The Lancet* (1991); 337:1197–200.

Sirtori, C. R. et al. "Soy and cholesterol reduction: clinical experience." *J Nutr* (1995). 125:598S–605S; *See also* Fiber, Phytoestrogens.

SPINACH

Kelsay, J. L. et al. "Mineral balances of men fed a diet containing fiber in fruits and vegetables and oxalic acid in spinach for six weeks." *J Nutr* (1988); 118(10):1197–2010. *See also* Antioxidants, Cruciferous vegetables, Other special properties.

SUNFLOWER

See Antioxidants.

SWEET POTATO

See Antioxidants.

TEA

Many studies, i.e.

Akinyanja et al. "Association of serum lipids with coffee, tea and egg consumption in free-living subjects." *Nature* (1967); 214:426–7.

Chung, S. Y. et al. "Tea and cancer". (review). *J Nat Cancer Inst* (1993); 85(13):1038–49. Dept. of Food and Nutrition, University of Shizuoka, Japan.

Green and Jucha. "Effect of coffee and tea on serum lipids in the rat." *J Epidemiol Commun* (1986); 40:324–9.

Lou, F. Q. et al. "A study on tea pigment in the prevention of atherosclerosis." Zhejing Medical Univ. Hospital, Hangzhou, China.

Nakayama, M. et al. "Inhibition of influenza virus infection by tea." Letters in *App Microbio* (1990); 11:38–40.

Yukihiko, H. "The effects of tea polyphenols on cardiovascular diseases." Food Research Labs., Mitsui Norin Co Ltd., Fujieda City, Shizuka Prefecture 426, Japan. *See also* Flavonoids.

TOMATO

See Antioxidants.

WALNUT

2 large-scale studies, i.e.

Fraser, G. E. et al. "A possible protective effect of nut consumption on risk of coronary heart disease: the Adventist Health Study." *Arch Intern Med* (1992); 152:1416–24.

Sabata, J. et al. "Effects of walnuts on serum lipid levels and blood pressure in normal men." *NE J Med* (1993); 328:603–7. *See also* Essential fatty acids.

WATERCRESS

Fairweather-Tait, S. J. et al. "Studies on calcium absorption from milk using a double label stable isotope method." *BJ Nutr* (1989); 62:379–88.

Messegue, M. *Health Secrets of Plants and Herbs*. Pan, London, 1981.

Vogel, Dr. A. *The Nature Doctor*. Vogel, Switzerland, 1952. *See also* Antioxidants, Lettuce & salad greens, Other special properties.

WHEAT GERM

See Antioxidants, Essential fatty acids.

WHEAT, RICE & WHOLE GRAINS

Leathwood, P. et al. "Effects of slow release carbohydrates in the form of bean flakes on the evolution of hunger and satiety in man." *Appetite* (1988); 10:1–11. *See also* Fiber, Phytoestrogens.

WINTER SQUASH

See Antioxidants, Other special properties.

YOGURT

Many studies, i.e.

Brassart, D. et al. "The selection of dairy bacterial strains with probiotic properties based on their adhesion to human intestinal epithelial cells." Nestlé Research Centre, Lausanne, Switzerland.

Gotz, V. P. et al. "Prophylaxis against ampicillin-associated diarrhea with a lactobacillus preparation." *Am J Hosp Pharm* (1979); 35:754–7.

Halpern, G. M. et al. "Influence of long-term yoghurt consumption in young adults." *Int J Immuno-ther* (1991); VII(4):205–10.

Hilton, E. et al. "Ingestion of yogurt containing *Lactobacillus acidophilus* as prophylaxis for candidal vaginitis." *Ann Int Med* (1992); 116:353–357.

Marks, J. "Gut flora and health: current status and future prospects." Review presented at *Gut Flora and Health Conference*, Yakult UK, London, 1996.

Niv, M. et al. "Yogurt in the treatment of infantile diarrhea." *Clinical Pediatrics* (1963); 7:407–10.

Siitonen, S. et al. "Effect of lactobacillus GG yoghurt in prevention of antibiotic associated diarrhoea." *Ann Med* (1990); 22:57–59.

Wynckel, A. et al. "Intestinal absorption of calcium from yoghurt in lactase-deficient subjects." *Reprod Nutr Dev* (1991); 31:411–18.

INDEX

Page numbers in **bold** refer to main entries in the *Food profiles* section. Page numbers in *italics* indicate recipes.

YZ

ACKNOWLEDGMENTS

AUTHOR'S ACKNOWLEDGMENTS
I would like to thank James W. B. Richmond for his great help with research. My gratitude also goes to the many people who have helped me locate information, especially Dr. Alan Long.

DK PUBLISHING
would like to thank Sara Harper and Nicola Graimes for editorial help; Clare Marshall and Johnny Pau for design assistance; Berit Vinegrad for preparing the dishes that appear throughout the book; Valerie Barret for help with the recipe section; Sue Bosanko for the index; Jasmine Challis for the nutritional analysis in the recipe section.

ILLUSTRATORS
Laura Jackson: symbols throughout *Food Profiles*, pp. 30–73.
Mick Gillah and Tony Graham: digestion illustration, p. 24.
Lorraine Harrison: illustrations throughout *Improving Your Health*, pp. 76–93.

PICTURE CREDITS
All photography by Steve Gorton and Andy Crawford except for: Science Photo Library/John Mead: p. 9 top left, p. 14 bottom right; British Museum, Bridgeman Art Library/John White: p. 10 bottom left; Arkopharma, France: p. 11 top right; Science Photo Library/John Mead: p. 14 bottom center; Food photography pp. 12–13; 46; 49; 98–141 Andrew Whittuck.

NUTRITIONAL DATA
The *Food Profiles* pp. 30–73 contain nutritional data from *The Composition of Foods*. It is reproduced with the permission of the Royal Society of Chemistry and the Controller of Her Majesty's Stationery Office.

NUTRITIONAL ANALYSIS
All nutritional analysis figures are approximate and are based on figures from the tables in *The Composition of Foods* (with additional data for manufactured and other products where appropriate), not by direct analysis of prepared dishes. Because the level and availability of nutrients varies, both in natural ingredients and in manufactured products, the figures are intended as a guide and not as an absolute amount.

If salt is given as a measured amount within a recipe, it has been included in the nutritional analysis for sodium. If a recipe's instructions say "season to taste," salt has not been included in the nutritional analysis for sodium. Seasoning to taste can result in widely varying levels of sodium, because each cook will have their own views about the amount of salt to use in a recipe.

Fried food may also vary in its fat content, depending on factors such as the initial temperature of the fat when food is added and the temperature of the fat during frying. The figure for total fat includes not only fatty acids (both saturated and unsaturated) but also other nonfatty material, such as phospholipids and sterols.

The amount and composition of salad dressings vary widely. Salad dressing is only included in nutritional analysis of recipes that specify dressing quantity and ingredients.